Pulmonary Tuberculosis
A Journey down the Centuries

The captain of all these men of death that came against him to take him away, was the Consumption, for it was that that brought him down to the grave.

John Bunyan *The Life and Death of Mr Badman*

The student who dates his knowledge of tuberculosis from Koch may have a very correct but a very incomplete, appreciation of the subject.

Sir William Osler

Pulmonary Tuberculosis

A Journey down the Centuries

R. Y. Keers

MD, FRCP Ed, FRCP Glasg, FRSE

Late Consultant Chest Physician, North
Staffordshire Hospital Centre,
Formerly Medical Director, Red Cross Sanatoria
of Scotland, and
Honorary Consultant in Diseases of the Chest
to the Army in Scotland

Foreword by
Sir John Crofton

MA, MD, FRCP Ed, FRCP Lond

Professor of Respiratory Diseases and
Tuberculosis, University of Edinburgh

Baillière Tindall · London

A BAILLIÈRE TINDALL book
published by Cassell Ltd
35 Red Lion Square, London WC1R 4SG
and at Sydney, Auckland, Toronto, Johannesburg
an affiliate of
Macmillan Publishing Co. Inc.
New York

© 1978   Baillière Tindall
a division of Cassell Ltd

First published 1978

ISBN 0 7020 0679 3

Designed by Peter Powell
Printed in Great Britain at
The Spottiswoode Ballantyne Press by
William Clowes & Sons Limited,
London, Colchester and Beccles

British Library Cataloguing in Publication Data

Keers, Robert Young
Pulmonary tuberculosis, a journey down the centuries.
1. Tuberculosis—History
I. Title
616.2'46'0609   RC310

ISBN 0-7020-0679-3

Contents

Foreword

Tuberculosis is known to have been one of the oldest of human
diseases, since its effects on bones can be identified. We do not
know how prevalent it may have been in ancient times but we do
know how disastrously it spread in Europe in the eighteenth and
nineteenth centuries when an important percentage of all deaths
were due to it. Though not raging with the brief and dramatic fury
of bubonic plague or cholera, which spread such panic in societies
all over the world, tuberculosis was the perpetual spectre in the
background. It carried off the young, the beautiful and the talented,
and indeed many others who were none of these but who found it
just as unpleasant to die and to suffer the grim cat-and-mouse
sequence of temporary improvement followed by tragic relapse.
No one knew when it would strike. Whole families might be
devastated. No wonder it was grimly promoted 'The Captain of all
these Men of Death' by John Bunyan.

Few diseases have had such extensive or such long continued
impact on the consciousness of mankind. In few has there been such
a dramatic reversal of dread as when, for the first time, truly effective
remedies appeared on the scene some three decades ago. In a few
years the outlook for individual patients was transformed. In a little
longer there was a steep fall in attack-rate. In countries which had
the knowledge, the money and the men, the Captain of the Men of
Death was soon demoted and listed for ignominious retirement,
though alas most of the poorer countries lagged, and still lag, sadly
behind.

Dr Keers, who was himself a distinguished specialist in the field
and a much sought-after teacher of young men, traces in this book
the long story of pulmonary tuberculosis from its earliest history to
the present day. He describes century after century of fumbling even
for a definition and identification of the disease as one entity; the

gradual elucidation of its manifestations; the dramatic discovery by Koch of its cause; the further long latent period before that discovery led to the evolution of an effective remedy; the fight-back by the bacillus with drug resistance; the discovery of further drugs and their combination to prevent resistance, and the final triumphant application of these methods to abolish this age-old threat to mankind, at least in those countries sufficiently rich and sufficiently organized to meet that threat. An enormous challenge still remains, a challenge to develop methods of prevention and treatment cheap enough and easy enough to be used on a mass scale in the poorer countries of Asia, Africa and South America. Devoted people are working on that task, but much is still to be done.

Any health worker or administrator who has ever had to deal with tuberculosis will find this book a fascinating and scholarly review of an entrancing story. But it should be of equal interest to the intelligent layman to read of the early millennial triumphs, and of the final ignominious exorcism, of one of the age-old spectres of society, now, after so many centuries, to haunt us no more.

JOHN CROFTON

February, 1978

Preface

Historical accounts of pulmonary tuberculosis have been written
previously and students of this aspect of the disease will be familiar
with the works of Flick, Pièry & Roshem, Webb and Lawrason
Brown, all of which have been freely consulted by the author. In
none of these is the story taken beyond the era of collapse therapy,
and the events of 1944, that *annus mirabilis*, have still to be recounted
and fitted into the long historical record. The object of this book is
to bring the record up-to-date but, lest in the euphoria of the
chemotherapy age anyone should be tempted to forget the herculean
labours of the past, the reader has been taken on a journey down the
centuries and has been introduced to those illustrious men who made
major contributions to the knowledge and understanding of what
was for so long the world's greatest killing disease. Those of us
whose acquaintance with tuberculosis began in the early 1930s have
witnessed a wonderful metamorphosis and now that it has become
possible to speak of the cure of tuberculosis without putting the word
cure in inverted commas we may be forgiven if we believe in our
hearts that the discovery of anti-tuberculosis chemotherapy
constituted the greatest medical miracle of the twentieth century.

The writing of this book would have been impossible without the
help of Miss J.P.S. Ferguson, MA, Librarian of the Royal College of
Physicians of Edinburgh, and her staff of skilled and patient library
assistants on whom a veritable barrage of queries and requests for
references descended. The brunt of this barrage was borne by Mrs
Mairi Lewis and every request was met with promptitude even when
it involved tracing the location of a rare volume outwith Great
Britain. Thanks to this efficient and courteous service the drafting of
the original manuscript was seldom interrupted.

The labour of composition was much lightened by the constant
encouragement which the writer received from his old friend and

former co-author, Dr Brian Rigden, whose enthusiasm and kindly perceptive criticism sustained him throughout. Dr Rigden read each section of the manuscript as it was completed and made many constructive suggestions which have greatly improved the quality of the end product.

The deciphering and typing of the script was carried out in her spare time by the writer's former secretary, Mrs Sylvia Gilbert, without whose expertise and care the task of preparing the book for publication would have been much more burdensome.

All these made major contributions to the work, but thanks are due also to Dr Christopher Clayson who supplied much firsthand information about Sir Robert Philip, to Mr J.H.A.C. Crawford who assisted by outlining the history and development of the Royal Victoria Hospital Tuberculosis Trust and to Dr A.E. Hugh who provided the clue which led to the tracing of Silvanus Thompson's memorable address to the Röntgen Society.

A special word of appreciation and thanks is due to Professor Sir John Crofton who, with his usual grace and generosity, has consented to provide an introductory foreword to the book.

The editorial staff of the publishers have been most helpful throughout and the author is grateful for their cooperation and for the advice which was so generously extended while the book was going through the press.

R.Y. KEERS

May, 1978

50, Garth Avenue
Surby
Port Erin
Isle of Man

Chapter One
Tuberculosis in Antiquity

The aptness of Thomas Carlyle's definition 'History is the essence of innumerable biographies'[1] is well illustrated by clinical tuberculosis. Begun in antiquity this story has continued down the centuries and, in unfolding, has created its own monuments, each marked by the name of a man whose flash of genius or whose dedication has helped to illuminate the way towards the ultimate goal—the conquest of the disease. Now that this goal has become attainable the time seems appropriate to attempt to tell the story in its entirety and, in so doing, to pay tribute to the memory of those whose work has made this dream possible and turned a hope into a certainty.

When and where the battle with the disease began remains a matter for conjecture but there is evidence that *Mycobacterium tuberculosis* must have preceded recorded history since Bartels described the changes of spinal tuberculosis in the skeleton of a neolithic man.[2] No further evidence linking the disease with the long prehistoric epoch emerged and its origins remained shrouded in mystery until about 4000 B.C. when, with the rise of the early civilizations, the gradual withdrawal of the veil began.

Among the first of these civilizations was that of the Sumerians, centred on Mesopotamia, in the fertile lands irrigated by the Tigris and the Euphrates. Amongst their achievements was the invention of writing, using cuneiform signs on tablets of stone and, although some of the tablets which have survived provide evidence of the existence of a Sumerian medical profession, they do not, unfortunately, yield any information about the diseases which were prevalent.

As their power declined that of Babylon arose where, between 1948 and 1905 B.C., an able and enlightened monarch, Hammurabi,

1   Carlyle, T. *Critical and Miscellaneous Essays*. Vol. ii On History.
2   Bartels, P. (1907) Tuberkulose (Wirbelkaries) in der jungeren Steinzeit. *Arch. Anthrop.* n.F., 6, 243.

ruled. He produced what has become the oldest code of laws in the world, the Code of Hammurabi, which engraved on a pillar of hard stone now rests in the Louvre. The Code covers many facets of Babylonian life setting out, amongst others, laws relating to property, to criminal offences, to marriage and to medical practice. These last, of great interest to medical historians in general, contain nothing which directly involves the historian of tuberculosis other than possibly that law which runs

> If a man take a wife and she becomes afflicted with disease and if he set his face to take another he may. His wife who is afflicted with the disease he shall not put away. She shall remain in the house which she has built and he shall maintain her as long as she lives.

This reference to what was clearly a chronic disease of considerable duration has led some authorities to suggest that it was tuberculosis.[3] Apart from the Code of Hammurabi nothing has survived to tell of the medical practice and customs of the period and the great kingdom crumbled into decay leaving little to testify to its glories save the ruins of its cities.

Further civilizations had arisen both in lands adjacent to Babylon and in others far to the eastward. In Egypt there is evidence that an organized system of government was in existence as early as 4000 B.C. and it was there that a method of recording time was introduced and also a system of pictorial writing from which an alphabet was later to evolve. New writing materials were invented and the convenience of papyrus as opposed to clay tablets led to the birth of literature. Many fragments of Egyptian medical papyri have come down to us and constitute the oldest medical documents extant. While these papyri were produced at a relatively late date they embody medico-magical knowledge and practice dating back to much earlier times and, although they cannot strictly speaking be regarded as medical treatises, they appear to contain extracts of medical passages from earlier prototypes which have never come to light. Among the best known and most complete of these is the Ebers papyrus discovered in 1862 in a tomb at Thebes by Professor Georg Ebers. This document contains, in addition to many spells and incantations, some 40 groups of recognizable remedies and prescriptions.

3 Flick, L. F. (1925) *Development of our Knowledge of Tuberculosis*. p. 9. Philadelphia: published by author.

The interpretation of the medical papyri has posed problems of great difficulty and it is possible that the precise pathology underlying some of the clinical conditions may never be determined. Certainly nothing has so far been found in these writings which can be accepted as providing convincing evidence of the existence of tuberculosis. Fortunately there is compensation for this lack of documentary evidence in valuable and authoritative findings stemming from two other sources. The first of these results from the predilection of Egyptian kings and nobles for keeping dwarfs, pygmies, hunchbacks and other malformed individuals in their households and it is to this idiosyncrasy that we are indebted for the numerous drawings and sculptures on the walls of tombs which have provided an instructive pathological picture gallery. Magicoreligious reasons demanded that any obvious bodily deformity be faithfully depicted and, since Egyptian artists excelled in craftsmanship and in fidelity to nature, the result has been some tomb portraits of hunchbacks in which the deformity is so accurately reproduced that a diagnosis of spinal tuberculosis can be made without hesitation.

The second source of authoritative information has been the examination of human remains. The Egyptian practice of mummification has conserved for modern investigation examples of Egypt's population from successive phases of history which endured for nearly 40 centuries and these have yielded much valuable data concerning the antiquity of certain diseases, particularly those involving the skeletal system. Clear evidence of lesions resulting from tuberculosis of bone has been found, dating back to the Early Dynastic period (*c.* 3400 B.C.), and conclusive proof of the existence of spinal tuberculosis in ancient Egypt came to light during the examination of the well-preserved mummy of a member of the 21st Dynasty priesthood of Amin, Nesperehan by name. Not only did examination show the characteristic deformity due to destruction and collapse of the thoracic vertebrae but there was, in addition, unmistakable evidence of an associated chronic psoas abscess.[4]

In contrast to the findings of the changes associated with skeletal tuberculosis no evidence has been forthcoming of visceral involvement and yet such lesions must almost certainly have co-existed. The lack of pathological proof of this point is understandable when the technique of Egyptian embalmers is considered. The process involved

4 Cave, A. J. E. (1939) The evidence for the incidence of tuberculosis in ancient Egypt. *Br. J. Tuberc.* 33, 142.

the extraction from the body cavity of all the viscera except the heart, and after extraction these were desiccated by exposure to heat before the application of the natron, oils and resins designed for their permanent preservation. The viscera were subsequently put together in four packages and entombed with the mummy but such a process of 'preservation' had made quite hopeless the quest for evidence of pre-existing pathological change.

Meanwhile in the east the Indo-Aryans had become another advanced civilization and have left medical records in Sanskrit, the earliest of which, the Rig-Veda which was written about 1500 B.C., suggests that they were acquainted with pulmonary tuberculosis. More positive evidence to this effect is forthcoming in a later series of works, the Ayur-Veda, dated about 700 B.C. which contains such *obiter dicta* as 'a consumptive who is evidently master of himself, who has a good digestion, is not emaciated and is at the beginning of the disease the physician can cure' and 'the physician who wants great fame cures a man attacked by consumption'.[5] Further study makes it clear that the symptoms of tuberculosis and, to a certain degree, the diagnosis were well understood. Treatment was largely based on hygiene and diet; residence at high altitudes, avoidance of fatigue and gentle horse-riding found favour, while milk, vegetables and a variety of meats including such delicacies as monkey meat, rats, snakes and earthworms were recommended. There is nothing in the Ayur-Veda to suggest that there was any suspicion of contagion, autopsies were not carried out and although the Laws of Manu, which are amongst the early Sanskrit writings (*c.* 1000 B.C.), declared that sufferers from tuberculosis were unclean and forbade Brahmins to marry into a family where the disease existed,[6] this ruling appears to have been a religious taboo rather than a measure of hygienic prophylaxis.

Still further to the east a Chinese civilization was groping for medical knowledge and the Emperor Shen Nung, reigning about 3000 B.C., had discovered a large number of drugs and poisons, many of them by the somewhat unorthodox procedure of self-experiment. This knowledge he incorporated into a text, Pen Tsao, the Chinese materia medica, which, in successive editions, was to be used in Chinese medicine for the next 5000 years. 'Lung fever' and 'lung

5 Webb, G. B. (1936) *Tuberculosis*. pp. 20–4. New York: P. B. Hoeber.
6 Brown, L. (1941) *Story of Clinical Pulmonary Tuberculosis,* p. 3. Baltimore: Williams & Wilkins.

4

cough', which must have included tuberculosis, were noted in ancient Chinese writings as far back as 2698 B.C.[7] with accompanying symptoms of emaciation, cough and the expectoration of blood and pus. It was appreciated that cure was difficult which probably explains the bizarre remedies advocated including the dung of animals and man, the urine of women and infants, the lungs of the hog and the ashes of hair.

While the study of the relics of antiquity has provided some evidence of the existence of tuberculosis, both in prehistoric times and amongst the oldest civilizations, it has told us little else. It is clear that, for all their familiarity with postmortem material which the technique of embalming involved, the Egyptians evinced little interest in anatomy or physiology nor were they particularly concerned to ascertain the cause of death. This is in striking contrast to the spirit of inquiry and the thirst for knowledge which was the hallmark of the civilization then arising in Greece which was to add immeasurably to the sum of human learning and was to provide the first of the great names which adorn the scroll of honour of tuberculosis. It is within this civilization of ancient Greece and amongst the islands of the Grecian archipelago that the history of tuberculosis really begins.

7   Hall, G. A. M., quoted by Meachen, G. N. (1936) *A Short History of Tuberculosis*. p. 1, London: John Bale, Sons & Danielsson.

Chapter Two
The Period of Clinical Observation and Deduction

The development of Greek medicine may be divided into three phases. The first concerns legends rather than history and presents the problem both of differentiating between fact and fantasy and of separating gods from men. Apollo was held to have taught the healing art to Chiron, the wisest of the centaurs, and he in turn instructed Aesculapius who later was to perform miracles of healing at Delphi. Whether or not Aesculapius had a human existence is uncertain. Some authorities consider it possible that he lived about 1250 B.C. and it is notable that, in the *Iliad*, Homer refers to the sons of Asklepios as 'the cunning leeches Podalarius and Machaon'. In the concluding phase of his life, however, fantasy displaces fact since the story goes that Pluto, the ruler of the underworld, fearing that the therapeutic success of Aesculapius threatened the supply of souls to his dominion, appealed to the supreme god Zeus who obligingly slew the offender with a thunderbolt.

This premature demise of Aesculapius was more than offset by his posthumous deification and ultimately he was worshipped at hundreds of temples or Asklepieia scattered through Greece. Chief amongst the worshippers were the sick who flocked there hoping to be healed through the ritual of temple sleep. This ritual involved an initial sacrificial offering, followed by a purifying bath, after which the patient composed himself to sleep in the long colonnades of the temple: during this sleep Aesculapius appeared to him in a dream, gave advice and treatment and in the morning he departed cured.

Our knowledge of the ritual of temple sleep is derived mainly from inscriptions on a series of stone tablets which were found at Epidauros, one of the most famous of the Asklepieia. The tablets are in effect case records and they contain the histories of 44 patients, all of whom experienced immediate and miraculous cure. No instance of failure has been recorded and death is never mentioned. In none of these cited cases are the symptoms in any way suggestive of tuberculosis but this is, perhaps, hardly surprising in view of the high degree of selectivity which was apparently practised in record keeping, allied to the prognosis of tuberculosis at that period as described later in the writings of the Hippocratic School. Although initially the regimen at the Asklepieia was dominated by the mystical and the supernatural, a more rational approach is apparent later with increasing emphasis being laid on the importance of diet, bathing and exercise. Physical treatment came to replace the overnight miracle and patients stayed at the Asklepieia for days or weeks.

While patients continued to flock to the Asklepieia Greek medicine approached the second phase in its development in the era of the early Greek philosophers. They refused to be guided solely by a belief in the supernatural and encouraged men to seek out for themselves the causes and reasons for all the phenomena of nature. Pythagoras and his pupil Alcmaeon, living about 500 B.C., may be said to have determined the empirical course which Greek medicine was to take in the hands of Hippocrates and his followers who dominated the third phase of its development and who were the initiators of a primitive form of scientific medicine, the forerunner of medicine as we know it today.

Hippocrates is thought to have lived from about 460 B.C. to 375 B.C. and is said to have been born on the island of Cos close to the coast of Asia Minor and, although he is known to have travelled fairly extensively and to have practised both in Thessaly and Athens, it is with his birthplace and with the school of medicine established there that his name is forever linked. While relatively little is known about Hippocrates the man a very complete account of his teaching and his methods is available in the books of the Hippocratic Collection. This remarkable collection comprises one hundred or more books although only a proportion of these are considered to have been written by Hippocrates himself. Much scholarly research and argument has been devoted to determining which of the volumes are his own, nevertheless the inspiration for them came from Hippocrates and the methods which they describe are those which he taught.

> To him medicine owes the art of clinical inspection and observation and he is above all the exemplar of that flexible, critical well-poised attitude of mind ever on the lookout for sources of error which is the very essence of the scientific spirit.[1]

1 Garrison, F. H. (1917) *An Introduction to the History of Medicine*. p. 82. Philadelphia: Saunders.

It is to the Hippocratic Collection that one turns for the first authentic account of clinical tuberculosis. Scattered throughout the volumes are numerous references to phthisis, the term which the Greeks introduced to describe disease accompanied by progressive weight loss but which subsequently came to denote a special type of phthisis associated with pulmonary symptoms. By careful correlation of these scattered references, some of them quite fragmentary, it is possible to obtain a fairly clear-cut picture of the observations of the Hippocratic School, of their interpretation of these observations and hence of the extent of their knowledge of tuberculosis. Most forms of the disease appear to have been seen by them but they did not recognize its unity nor had they any real appreciation of the associated pathological changes. This serious defect in their learning arose from the lack of postmortem studies for, until the advent of the Alexandrian school of medicine, the Greeks performed no autopsies and it is considered unlikely that Hippocrates ever actually saw a tuberculous human lung.[2] The word 'tubercle', which does appear in some of the texts, was applied to any nodule wherever situated and of whatever aetiology while the word 'phyma', which is frequently encountered, bore a similar meaning. It is quite clear that these terms carried no specific connotation, such as that which later linked the tubercle to tuberculous disease, and it is believed that the Hippocratic concept of the pathology of phthisis was based on the appearances noted in animal tissues together with the study of external manifestations of the disease. A passage taken from the work *On Internal Affections* in the Collection speaks of dropsy 'connected with tubercles of the lung which get filled up with water and burst into the chest'. In support of this statement the writer refers to observations made on cattle, sheep and swine which are said 'to be very subject to these tubercles (phymata)' and he argues that man is still more liable, adding that in many cases 'Empyema originates in tubercles.'[3]

This lack of understanding of the basic pathology was reflected in their ideas on pathogenesis. Their main theory postulated defluxions proceeding from the head which on reaching the lungs set up phthisis or empyema while, should they reach the spine, 'another species of phthisis' was produced.[4] Contagion is not mentioned in any of the

2   Webb, G. B. (1936) *Tuberculosis*. p. 49. New York: P. B. Hoeber.
3   Adams, F. (1849) *The Genuine Works of Hippocrates*. (Trans) i, p. 88. London: Sydenham Society.
4   *Ibid*. p. 76

Hippocratic writings but reference is made to the possibility of phthisis being hereditary, as in the case of the daughter of Euryanax;[5] such a possibility was regarded as adding greatly to the difficulty of the problem.

The shortcomings of the Greeks in the field of pathology can be forgiven and forgotten in the light of their clinical observations on phthisis which are masterly pieces of descriptive writing, covering every point of importance. The cardinal symptoms, the age incidence, the seasonal variation and the prognosis (the latter, unfortunately, almost invariably poor) are all discussed in one or other of the volumes. Their diagnosis was based almost entirely on semeiology coupled with the meticulous and painstaking observation of external features, though there are occasional passages in the Collection which suggest that a limited degree of physical examination must have been attempted. Thus there are several references to râles 'by which the existence of matter in the lungs is ascertained'[6] while the value of succussion in the localization of empyema is mentioned repeatedly, one such passage stating that 'empyema forms in phthisical persons and that in their case, too, a sound like that of water in a bladder may be heard on succussion'.[7] There is yet one further familiar sign recorded, namely, a sound like that made by new leather, which is heard in pleurisy on applying the ear directly to the chest wall.[8] It is quite clear that throughout the Collection the authors have great difficulty in separating tuberculosis from other chronic respiratory illnesses, particularly empyema, but this in no way detracts from the brilliance of the clinical descriptions.

It is difficult to form even an approximate estimate of the prevalence of phthisis in the days of Hippocrates but a sufficiency of the clinical descriptions conform so closely to those of pulmonary tuberculosis as to suggest that the condition was seen frequently. Thus the opening paragraphs of Book I *Of the Epidemics* contain the following observations:

> Early in the beginning of spring and through the summer and towards winter, many of those who had been long gradually declining, took to bed with symptoms of phthisis; in many cases formerly of a doubtful character the disease then became confirmed; in these the constitution

5 *Ibid.* p. 394.
6 *Ibid.* p. 91.
7 *Ibid.* p. 76.
8 Finlayson, J. (1892) On Hippocrates. *Glasg. med. J. 37,* 267.

inclined to the phthisical. Many, and in fact, the most of them, died; and of those confined to bed I do not know if a single individual survived for any considerable time; they died more suddenly than is common in such cases.[9]

There is a ring of authority about this passage which suggests that the writer was only too familiar with the sequence of events which he is describing.

The treatment recommended by the Hippocratic School was, on the whole, rational. The regimen for the acute stage consisted of rest, baths, attention to the bowels and a liquid diet, while in the more chronic case mild exercise was permitted with a diet of rich easily digested food. Milk was used very liberally, human milk being regarded as the best followed by that of goats, asses and cows. Drugs were employed sparingly, mainly as purgatives or expectorants, while bleeding was reserved for the acute stage or for the relief of complications such as the pain of a pleurisy where the more usual treatment, the application of a poultice of toasted millet, had failed. More active measures were suggested for certain cases of empyema when it was recommended than an incision be made at

> the level of the third rib from the last and then make a perforation with a trocar so as to give vent to a small portion of the fluid; the opening is then to be filled with a tent, and the remainder evacuated after twelve days.[10]

No survey of the work and influence of Hippocrates is complete without reference to the Aphorisms, those distillates of clinical wisdom which are the most famous of all the writings. Certain of these refer to phthisis and those quoted here are taken from the translation prepared in 1849 by Francis Adams of Banchory, Kincardineshire, for the Sydenham Society.

Section III   No. 10. Autumn is a bad season for persons in consumption.

No. 13. If the summer be dry and northerly and the autumn rainy and southerly, headaches occur in winter, with coughs, hoarseness, coryzae and in some cases consumptions.

No. 22. Of autumn, most of the summer, quartan and irregular fever, enlarged spleen, dropsy, phthisis, strangury, lientery, dysentery, sciatica, quinsy,

9 Adams, F. (3) pp. 353–4.
10 *Ibid.* p. 88.

asthma, ileus, epilepsy, maniacal and melancholic disorders.

No. 29. To persons past boyhood haemoptysis, phthisis, acute fever, epilepsy, and other diseases, but especially the aforementioned.

Section IV No. 8. We must be guarded in purging phthisical persons upwards.

Section V No. 9. Phthisis most commonly occurs between the ages of eighteen and thirty-five years.

No. 11. In persons affected with phthisis, if the sputa which they cough up have a heavy smell when poured upon coals, and if the hairs of the head fall off, the case will prove fatal.

No. 13. In persons who cough up frothy blood, the discharge of it comes from the lungs.

No. 14. Diarrhoea attacking a person affected with phthisis is a mortal symptom.

No. 15. Persons who become affected with empyema after pleurisy, if they get clear of it in forty days from the breaking of it, escape the disease; but if not, it passes into phthisis.

Section VI No. 12. When a person has been cured of chronic haemorrhoids, unless one be left, there is danger of dropsy or phthisis supervening.

The epidemiology, the clinical features and the prognosis all receive attention in these succinct paragraphs which have stood for centuries as examples of the astute observation and sound common sense which characterized the work of the Hippocratic School and earned for it high honour in the annals of medical history.

In the period following the death of Hippocrates, which is believed to have occurred about 355 B.C., little new was added to the knowledge of tuberculosis. Aristotle (384–322 B.C.), although he was not a physician but a profound philosopher and the first great biologist, carried out extensive studies in comparative anatomy and left a description of scrofula seen in hogs.[11] He also commented on the possibility of contagion in phthisis, noting that persons in the proximity of consumptives tended to contract the disease. This, he suggested, was due to some disease-producing substance exhaled into the air in the patient's breath.[12]

11 Flick, L. F. (1925) *Development of our Knowledge of Tuberculosis*. pp. 72–3 Philadelphia: published by author.
12 Webb, G. B. (2) pp. 36–7.

Even the school of medicine founded in Alexandria in 332 B.C. is not noted for any progress in the study of tuberculosis although the Alexandrian teachers enjoyed the advantage, denied to their predecessors, of practising human dissection. It is possible, though, that their interest lay primarily in physiology rather than in morbid anatomy since, according to Celsus, prisoners were procured by royal permission and dissected alive, a procedure which he considered to be far the best method of attaining knowledge.[13] An alternative or additional explanation may lie in the fate of the vast library accumulated in the Alexandrian school which amounted to 700 000 volumes but which was wrecked and burnt at a time of civil tumult by a fanatical mob intent on sweeping away the old in order to establish the new. In the process most of the literary output from the school perished and our knowledge of it is derived mainly from the work of Celsus and Galen, particularly the writings of the former which have been regarded as a partial replacement for the lost literature of Alexandria.

Grecian medicine declined with their empire, the glories of Alexandria passed into history and gradually the centre of interest was transferred to Rome to which many Greek physicians emigrated. Here they found scope for their skills since the average Roman citizen considered that medicine as a profession was beneath his dignity and for a time its practice was left in the hands of Greeks and slaves, neither being held in high esteem.

Some of the earliest evidence of Roman acquaintance with tuberculosis is found in the writings of Pliny the Elder (A.D. 23–79) who, although not a physician, was a close observer of all natural phenomena and produced a 37 volume treatise on natural history to which he added some comments on contemporary medical thought. In these he provides prescriptions for the treatment of cough (wolf's lung boiled in wine, bear's blood mixed with honey, horse's saliva) and of haemoptysis (gelatine of hare's meat or stag's horn ground to powder, mixed with the earth of Samos and moistened with myrtle wine).[14] It is fair to add that, in addition to these pharmaceutical oddities, the Romans of Pliny's period believed that a change to a warm, dry climate was helpful in phthisis as was a generous diet with abundance of milk. Pliny himself advocated sea voyages for phthisis and

13 Guthrie, D. (1945) *A History of Medicine*. p. 64. London: Thomas Nelson.
14 Castiglioni, A. (1933) History of tuberculosis, *Med. Life 40*, 5.

haemoptysis, believing that the retching associated with sea sickness had a beneficial effect on the lungs.[15]

It is, however, to two Greek physicians that we owe practically all our knowledge of tuberculosis as it appeared in the heyday of the Roman Empire. Aretaeus the Cappadocian is known only by his writings; nothing is known of the man himself and even the exact period in which he lived is uncertain although Adams[16] deduces from indirect evidence that it must have been about the middle of the second century A.D. His descriptions of diseases are unsurpassed for accuracy and are even more comprehensive than those of Hippocrates. In his chapter on phthisis in his first book *On the Causes and Symptoms of Chronic Diseases* the description of the advanced case of tuberculosis is a classic and merits quotation.

> Voice hoarse; neck slightly bent, tender, not flexible, somewhat extended; fingers slender, but joints thick; of the bones alone the figure remains, for the fleshy parts are wasted; the nails of the fingers crooked, their pulps are shrivelled and flat, for, owing to the loss of flesh, they neither retain their tension nor rotundity; and, owing to the same cause, the nails are bent, namely, because it is the compact flesh at their points which is intended as a support to them; and the tension thereof is like that of the solids. Nose sharp, slender; cheeks prominent and red; eyes hollow, brilliant and glittering; swollen, pale or livid in the countenance; the slender parts of the jaw rest on the teeth, as if smiling; otherwise of a cadaverous aspect. So also in all other respects, slender, without flesh; the muscles of the arms imperceptible; not a vestige of the mammae, the nipples only to be seen; one may not only count the ribs themselves, but also easily trace them to their terminations; for even the articulations at the vertebrae are quite visible; and their connections with the sternum are also manifest; the intercostal spaces are hollow and rhomboidal, agreeably to the configuration of the bone; hypochondriac region lank and retracted; the abdomen and flanks contiguous to the spine. Joints clearly developed, prominent, devoid of flesh, so also with the tibia, ischium and humerus; the spine of the vertebrae formerly hollow, now protrudes, the muscles on either side being wasted; the whole shoulder-blades apparent like the wings of birds. If in these cases disorder of the bowels supervene, they are in a hopeless state.[17]

Apart from this vivid word picture Aretaeus drew attention to evening fever, sweating and lassitude as clinical accompaniments of

15   Webb, G. B. (2) pp. 142–3.
16   Adams, F. (1856) *The Extant Works of Aretaeus*. (Trans) p. viii. London: Sydenham Society.
17   *Ibid.* pp. 310–11.

the disease and suggested also that simple inspection of the sputum
was of greater diagnostic value than testing it with fire or water.

He wrote on the treatment of phthisis in a chapter from *On the Cure
of Chronic Diseases*. It is unfortunate that part of the original text of
this chapter is missing but sufficient has survived to show that
Aretaeus, like Pliny, favoured a sea voyage and also believed strongly
in the value of milk: 'if one, then, will only drink plenty of this, he
will not stand in need of anything else'. Additional foods mentioned
are porridge, pastry and 'other edibles prepared with milk'.[18] Another
chapter of interest is that *On Persons affected with Empyema*, which is
followed by a short chapter *On Abscess in the Lung*.[19] It is clear that he
did not regard every case of pulmonary disease as phthisis and in
these chapters he has tried to set out criteria for differential diagnosis.
In so doing he achieved a degree of success which is quite remarkable
for that time.

While few biographical details are known about Aretaeus there is
information in abundance concerning the other great Greek physician
of the same period, Galen the Pergamite, a man who was not notably
given to reticence. Born at Pergamos in Asia Minor about A.D. 131,
the son of an architect, he received an education in philosophy at
Pergamos and Smyrna, and subsequently in medicine at Alexandria.
On leaving Alexandria he travelled in Greece, Italy and Palestine,
eventually returning to Pergamos where he was appointed surgeon
to the school of gladiators. He held this appointment for four years,
but not being particularly attracted to the practice of surgery[20] he left
for Rome in search of fame and fortune, both of which readily came
his way. He built up an extensive practice as a physician, acquired a
reputation as an experimental physiologist and was a voluminous
writer to whom some 500 books are attributed although only about
80 of these remain extant. He recognized the value of anatomy as a
basic science and studied it intensively but, unfortunately, dissection
of the human body had remained illegal in Rome so that his anatomical
researches were perforce carried out on apes and pigs. Galen unhesitatingly transferred his veterinary findings to human anatomy
and in so doing perpetrated many errors; errors which were only
corrected after the lapse of centuries.

Galen's approach to clinical tuberculosis, like that of his pre-

18 *Ibid.* pp. 478–9.
19 *Ibid.* pp. 312–16.
20 Finlayson, J. (1892) Galen., *Br. med. J.* 573.

decessors, had no basis of pathology and to him pulmonary phthisis arose from ulceration of the lung which might be due to trauma, to the extension of inflammation from the nose or throat or even to chilling of the lung. The majority of his recorded cases were associated with haemoptysis, which he considered to be pathognomonic of the disease, while amongst other common symptoms and signs he included chest pain, cough, sputum, hoarseness, fever and wasting.[21] He insisted that pulmonary ulceration was curable only in its early stages and regarded the earliest case as that seen after an initial haemoptysis and before the onset of cough. When a cough was accompanied by purulent sputum and fever had appeared, he held that the chances of a successful cure were greatly diminished. He believed that phthisis was contagious and considered it dangerous to live with patients who had consumption.[22]

His treatment consisted essentially of rest, restraint of cough and, in the initial stages, a ban on visitors to eliminate the strain of conversation. Diet occupied a prominent place in his regimen and he wrote about this subject in great detail, discussing the particular virtues of each variety of meat, fish and poultry. He was an enthusiast for milk which he held to be a specific in pulmonary ulceration providing that it be drunk as fresh as possible. He held the view that pulmonary ulceration demanded therapy similar to that employed to heal ulcers on the body surface but, since the medication could only reach the pulmonary lesion via the stomach, the remedies had either to be stronger or administered in larger dosage than for superficial foci. He favoured astringents obtained from plants, such as the pomegranate, which contained tannic acid and these, mixed with honey, were employed both as mixtures and as gargles. Plasters were applied to the chest, the most highly recommended being one which contained a lead salt and copper sulphate in a vehicle of lard and olive oil. When a cough was violent, and disturbing sleep, hyoscyamus seeds and the root of black mandrake were prescribed in a mixture which also contained opium and rhubarb though as a general rule, Galen was opposed to the use of narcotic drugs other than for the relief of a violent cough or severe pain.

It is unfortunate that Galen, unlike Hippocrates, has left no good accounts of clinical cases but only of miraculous cures. Furthermore

21 Walsh, J. (1931) Galen's treatment of pulmonary tuberculosis. *Am. Rev. Tuberc. pulm. Dis., 24, 1.*
22 *Ibid. 24, 36.*

he attempted to explain everything in the light of pure theory, thus substituting a pragmatic system of medical philosophy for the simple observation and interpretation of facts as taught by Hippocrates. Forceful, dogmatic and completely unimpeded by any sense of modesty, he acquired a reputation for infallability which remained intact long after his death, causing him to be regarded as the undisputed authority from whom none dared to differ. As a result medicine remained stagnant for nearly 14 centuries until the dead hand of Galen was removed from the tiller of progress by the work of Vesalius who dispelled many of the anatomical myths which had been created.

The authority and imperial might of Rome had begun to crumble but the final dissolution was delayed by the expedient of the Emperor Constantine in transferring his capital from Rome to Byzantium in A.D. 330. This inaugurated the epoch of Byzantine medicine, in which little new was added to existing knowledge though the Byzantine physicians did collect and transcribe much of the work of their predecessors which might otherwise have been lost. Alexander of Tralles (A.D. 525 to 605), one of the few whose writings are regarded as showing any originality, left an excellent clinical description of pleurisy which is among the classics of medicine.[23] The last physician of the classical school, Paul of Aegina, who produced his Epitome, consisting of seven books on medicine and surgery, merely reiterated the views of Galen on phthisis and added nothing new.[24]

After the final collapse of the Roman Empire in the sixth century the period known as the 'Dark Ages' unfolded, a period which was to span a 1000 years during which 'learning was no longer held in high esteem, experiment was discouraged and originality was a dangerous asset'.[25] The practice of medicine passed mainly into the hands of two vastly different groups, the Christian Church and the Arab scholars, and it is necessary to consider how each of these groups dealt with the problems with which they were faced and in particular tuberculosis.

The initial influence of the early Christian Church on medical science was wholly retrograde, the result in part of a too literal interpretation of its Founder's instruction to His followers to heal the

23 Guthrie, D. (13) p. 80.
24 Adams, F. (1844–7) *The Seven Books of Paulus Aegineta*. (Trans) London: Sydenham Society.
25 Guthrie, D. (13) p. 84.

sick. This led to a denial to physicians of the power of healing and to the exaltation of prayer and fasting above all other remedies. A further difficulty was created by the Church's view of the aetiology of disease which in many instances was regarded as a punishment for sin, with prayer and repentance again the sole prescription. The human body was held to be sacred and its dissection remained a crime so that anatomy and physiology continued as dead sciences to be studied only in the pages of Galen. It was in truth a grim and desolate period until ultimately a gleam of light appeared with the gradual emergence of monastic medicine. St Benedict of Nursia had laid it down that the care of the sick should be one of the main objectives of the order which he founded and, little by little, the monasteries began to take increasing responsibility for tending the sick poor for whose reception a hospice might be created within the monastery confines and for whose use a herb garden for the growing of medicinal herbs might be planted. Higher authorities in the order also believed that some time should be set aside for study and they encouraged, in particular, the collection and copying of the manuscript works of the great Greek physicians, which were thus preserved for dissemination when the Renaissance brought the invention of printing in its train.

The Arab physicians, so designated because they shared a common language, included Syrians, Persians and Spaniards. They likewise copied the Greek texts, were denied the right of human dissection and, apart from developments in chemistry and pharmacology they produced little that was original. Rhazes, held to be one of their greatest physicians, adhered to the views of Galen on phthisis while Avicenna, in his *Canon of Medicine,* considered it to be a general disease with local manifestations in the form of lung ulcers. He believed that it was contagious and he employed in treatment an intratracheal injection of an infusion of red roses and honey.[26]

Baghdad was sacked by the Mongols in 1236, the lands of Islam no longer provided the tranquillity desirable for study and so the centre of medical thought was switched westward to Salerno, site of the first organized medical school in Europe, where learning had been established on a sound basis. While the exact origins of the Salerno school are obscure it is believed to have reached the zenith of its fame in the eleventh century. Its most famous literary product was the *Regimen Sanitatis Salernitanum,* a work in verse of composite author-

26 Brown, L. (1941) *The Story of Clinical Pulmonary Tuberculosis.* p. 8. Baltimore: Williams & Wilkins.

ship and uncertain date which embodied much of the teaching of the school in a presentation popular enough to ensure for it a wide circulation. It contained some discussion on the care of the tuberculous patient but did not deviate in any significant respect from the teaching of Galen.

The school of Salerno eventually gave place to that of Montpellier where Arnold of Villanova (1235–1312), one of its earliest and most famous professors, taught that the pulmonary ulcers of phthisis were caused by cold humours falling drop by drop from the head and thus wearing away the lung,[27] whilst among the aphorisms for which he was noted appears the following:

> In most cases of scrofula external applications are better than the use of the knife. Scrofulous patients always have other sources of infection within them and so it does them no good to operate externally.[28]

—a truth which surgeons failed to appreciate for another 700 years.

The incidence of tuberculosis in Europe throughout the medieval period can only be a matter of conjecture. A rough indication expressed in figures may be found in the history of the ceremony of touching for 'The King's Evil'. The belief in the royal power to heal dated back to the time of Clovis the Frank (A.D. 496) and although initially the healing touch was extended to all manner of diseases it very shortly became restricted to scrofula, a term which covered various forms of non-pulmonary tuberculosis but which was applied chiefly to tuberculosis of the neck glands. Royal records of the period show that Edward I (1272–1307) touched 533 in one month while Philip of Valois (1328 to 1350) is credited with 1500 at a single ceremony.[29] Such figures suggest an appreciable and increasing incidence of this one manifestation of tuberculous disease from which one may reasonably deduce that the incidence of the pulmonary form was considerably higher.

The medical schools at Salerno and Montpelier had shone out like beacons in the otherwise unrelieved gloom of the remainder of medieval medicine which had then sunk to its lowest ebb with diagnosis based upon the position of the stars and the appearances of the urine. Treatment was either in the hands of the monks who used herbal remedies, the action of which they did not understand, and

27 Piery, M & Roshem, J. (1931) *Histoire de la Tuberculose*. pp. 41–2. Paris: Doin et Cie.
28 Webb, G. B. (2) p. 55.
29 *Ibid*. p. 30.

enjoined the sick to emulate the saints in their capacity for the endurance of suffering, or else the patient fell a prey to the itinerant quacks and ignorant humbugs of whom there was no lack.

It required the wonderful phenomenon of the Renaissance to enable men to throw off the tyranny of scholastic dogmatism, to break the stranglehold of the Church and to restore to learning and the pursuit of knowledge the position of honour and prestige with which they had been endowed in the civilizations of Greece and Rome.

Chapter Three
The Period of Anatomical and Pathological Study

The dawn of the Renaissance had been marked by the timely invention of printing and the year 1478 saw the publication in Florence of the works of Celsus. By the middle of the sixteenth century most of the great Greek texts had been translated into Latin and published.

A mutually beneficial alliance between the artists and the anatomists had resulted in a gradual easing of the restriction on dissection which left the way clear for the work of Andreas Vesalius (1514–1564) —the greatest anatomist of the Renaissance if not of all time. Appointed professor of anatomy at Padua he produced in 1543 his great work *De Humani Corporis Fabrica*, in which many of the errors perpetrated and perpetuated by Galen were corrected in the text and with which modern anatomy may be said to have begun. The principle of dissection having been established it was but logical that its objective should be extended to include something more than the mere acquisition of anatomical knowledge. Antonio Benivieni (?–1502) claimed that post-mortem examination was essential to find the hidden causes of disease[1] but there was a time lag of a century before Theophile Bonet in 1679 produced his *Sepulchretum* containing the results of autopsies during the sixteenth and seventeenth centuries. In the section *De Tabe in genere et pulmonari* some 46 autopsies were reported, together with an account of the symptoms which had preceded death. The collection included some of the cases of Jean Fernel (1497–1558), the leading Parisian physician of the day, who had described cavities (*vomicae*) in the lungs and had expressed the view that in consumptives these were of frequent occurrence.[2]

In the meantime other events were taking place and other ideas germinating. Philippus Aureolus Theophrastus Bombastus von Hohenheim, more commonly known as Paracelsus (1490–1541), had

1 Webb, G. B. (1936) *Tuberculosis*. p. 56. New York: P. B. Hoeber.
2 *Ibid*. pp. 56–7.

erupted on to the scene and had introduced a new dimension into medical controversy by prefixing his lectures with a public burning of the works of Galen. He remained a stormy petrel throughout his life but he was undoubtedly one of the outstanding physicians of the sixteenth century. He travelled widely in Europe, is known to have visited the tin mines in Cornwall and wrote a monograph on miners' phthisis which was published in 1567, 27 years after his death.[3] The monograph was based largely on his observations in the Fuger lead mines in the Tyrol and, with its description of miners' phthisis and of the effects of choke-damp, it must rank as one of the few original contributions of the period to clinical medicine.

A most notable event took place in 1546 when Heironymous Frascatorius (1483–1553) produced his major work *De Contagione* in which he described the three methods of infection: infection by direct contact, infection by fomites (he was the first to apply this term to infected clothing and utensils) and infection at a distance, as in plague. He postulated the existence of imperceptible particles or 'seminaria', the seeds of disease, which he believed could exist outside the body for several years and still infect. In phthisis he considered that the 'seminaria' could not only come from without but could also arise within the body from putrefaction of the humours.[4] He pondered on the possibility of destroying the 'seminaria' within the lungs and for a time considered the use of caustics, an idea which he ultimately rejected as posing too great a danger to the tissues. He believed in the prescription of expectorants and of arsenic and advised strongly against anything which might impede expectoration.[5] His ideas on infection found little acceptance at that time and more than a century was to elapse before any practical use was made of these enlightened views which entitle Frascatorius to be regarded as the founder of modern epidemiology.

Over the succeeding one hundred years nothing new was added to the knowledge of tuberculosis despite its prevalence in Europe. In Britain while actual statistics are lacking, there are sufficient references in Shakespeare's plays to provide evidence of popular familiarity with the disease. In *Much Ado about Nothing* Beatrice is made to take pity on her consumptive lover. We are further indebted to Shakespeare for his

3   Rosen, G. (1943) *History of Miners' Diseases: A Medical and Social Interpretation*. pp. 64–7. New York: Schuman.
4   Webb, G. B (1) pp. 37–8.
5   Castiglioni, A. (1933) History of tuberculosis. *Med. Life* N.S., *40*, 26.

most succinct and graphic description of pleural pain in the *The Tempest* Act I, Scene 2. 'Side-stitches that shall pen thy breath up.' Scrofula was common, the healing hand of royalty was much in demand and again Shakespeare shows in *Macbeth* Act IV, Scene 3 how well acquainted he was with the routine ceremonial of the procedure. Speculation as to the cause of phthisis was rife but despite the work of Frascatorius such speculation remained very wide of the mark. Any abnormality in the shape of the chest, whether developmental or acquired, was cited as a possible causative factor and Christopher Bennett (1617–1655) wrote in 1654 that deformed persons and those who had had limbs amputated were more liable to the disease than others.[6] In 1629 London bills of mortality began to specify the disease with 'consumption', 'feaver' and 'griping in the guts' as leading causes of death.[7]

Clearly the next step forward was overdue and it was taken eventually by Franciscus de le Boë (1614–1672) otherwise known as Sylvius who was professor of clinical and anatomical medicine at Leyden between 1648 and 1672. Anatomist, physiologist and chemist, he was also a truly great clinician and the first to introduce clinical instruction where the excellence of his teaching brought students flocking to his small infirmary of 12 beds. It was, however, his work in the field of morbid anatomy which brought him face to face with the problem of tuberculosis and it was he who associated the small hard nodules discovered in various tissues at autopsy and termed tubercles (a name applied to every small nodule, since the days of the Greeks) with the symptoms of phthisis from which the patient had suffered during life. He noted the tendency of the tubercles 'to grow in tissue and gradually to suppurate' and wrote concerning them 'I would not even hesitate to credit these tubercles with being the hereditary and fatal predisposition to consumption in certain families even though they are not encountered elsewhere in a form in which they can be outwardly recognised'.[8] The origin of these tubercles had to be explained and Sylvius expressed the view that they represented small lymph glands, so situated within the lung substance as to be normally invisible, which had undergone a degenerative change

6   Meachen, G. N. (1936) *A Short History of Tuberculosis*. p. 6. London: John Bale Sons & Danielsson.

7   Burke, R. M. (1955) *An Historical Chronology of Tuberculosis*. p. 14. Springfield, Illinois: C. C. Thomas.

8   Flick, L. F. (1925) *Development of Our Knowledge of Tuberculosis*. pp. 78–80. Philadelphia: published by author.

which he considered analogous to that observed in the neck glands of scrofula. This view was erroneous and Bulloch was later to claim that the error hampered progress for the succeeding hundred years[9] a verdict which may be considered harsh when applied to the man who was the first to link the tubercle so firmly with phthisis and to see an association between phthisis and scrofula, a particular piece of insight which placed him years ahead of his time.

Sylvius also lent his authority to the doctrine of contagion in tuberculosis, writing that

> the air expired by consumptives having been brought close to the mouth and nose is drawn in and in this way offensive and irritating emanations are continuously carried from the affected party to others especially relatives and when these are finally infected with the same poison they also fall into phthisis.[10]

From Leyden the news of his work and of the suggested association between tubercles and phthisis spread quickly and stimulated fresh interest and research. There was indeed ample evidence of the need for such further study since the disease was now widespread. It is believed that in 1667 25 per cent of deaths in London were due to phthisis[11] while Charles II, during his reign from 1660 to 1682, is reputed to have bestowed the royal touch on no fewer than 92 102 scrofulous persons.[12]

Amongst those applying their minds to the problem of phthisis was a former student at Leyden, Thomas Willis (1621–1675) who had not only become a physician of distinction but was also the tenant of the Sedleian Chair of natural philosophy at Oxford. He embodied his observations on the disease in a special chapter of his book on the *Practice of Physick* which was published in London some nine years after his death. He was one of the first to question the accepted doctrine of the day, that a diagnosis of phthisis could not be sustained in the absence of pulmonary ulceration, when he wrote

> A Phthisis is usually defined to be a pining away of the whole body, taking its rise from an Ulcer in the Lungs. But less true: because I have opened the dead bodies of many that have died of this disease, in whom the

9 Bulloch, W. (1911) *Tracts*. Part 441, Article no. 9.
10 Flick, L. F. (8) p. 82.
11 Brownlee, J. (1918) An investigation into the epidemiology of phthisis in Great Britain and Ireland. *Med. Res. Comm.* p. 43.
12 Guthrie, D. (1945) *A History of Medicine.* p. 210. London: Thomas Nelson.

Lungs were free from any Ulcer, yet they were set about with little swellings, or stones, or sandy matter throughout the whole . . . wherefore a *Phthisis* is better defined, *That it is a withering away of the whole body arising from an ill formation of the Lungs.*[13]

This description suggests that Willis had seen cases of miliary tuberculosis as well as instances of chronic fibroid disease with minimal cavitation. Pursuing further the variations which he had noted in the pulmonary pathology he continued

> but sometimes it happens that there is one Ulcer or hole, or happily two, formed in the lungs and the sides grow callous round about so that the matter being there gathered together is not conveyed into the mass of blood, but is daily expectorated though in a vast plenty. They that are so affected, as if they had but an issue in the Lungs, although they cast up much Spittle and thick and yellow matter every morning and a little sometimes all day, yet otherwise they live well enough in health, they breath, eat and sleep well, are well in flesh, or at least remain in an indifferent habit of body, and frequently arrive to old age: insomuch that some are said to have been consumptive thirty or forty years, and to have prolonged the disease even unto the term of their life (for that cause not being shortened). And in the mean time others who cough and spit less, within a few months fall into a hectick feaver, and in a short while are hurried into their grave.[14]

Willis was obviously noting and recording the differing individual reactions to the disease with which succeeding generations of physicians were to become fully acquainted.

Close on the heels of Willis came Richard Morton (1637–1698) who, having been deprived of his living as vicar of Kinver in Staffordshire in 1662 owing to his refusal to subscribe to the Act of Uniformity, turned to medicine as his second career. It is not known with certainty where he obtained his early training although he is believed to have studied for a time at Leyden but it is known that he obtained his M.D. at Oxford in 1670, on the nomination of the Prince of Orange, thereafter setting up practice in London at Grey Friar's Court, Newgate Street. Morton's claim to fame rests on his monumental treatise *Phthisiologia*, dedicated to his erstwhile patron William III and published in 1688. This was by far the most ambitious publication on the subject yet attempted and it set out admirably and at length con-

13 Willis, T. (1684) *Practice of Physick*. Phar II, Sect. I, Ch. VI. p. 28. London.
14 *Ibid.* p. 30.

temporary thought and opinion. Morton approached the subject by interpreting the word 'phthisis' in its most literal sense, namely a wasting of the body from any cause. He divided his work into three sections, the first dealing with wasting in general, the second with wasting from a consumption of the lungs and the third with wasting due to a symptomatic consumption of the lungs by which he implied a consumption of the lungs caused by and depending on some other preceding disease. As examples of such diseases he cited amongst others smallpox, measles, scarlet fever, pleurisy and diabetes.

It is clear that Morton had very extensive clinical experience and that he had also observed at autopsy virtually all the macroscopic appearances which one might expect to encounter in pulmonary tuberculosis. On occasions he misinterpreted his findings but in so doing he merely followed the theory of the times. His clinical observations and descriptions throughout remained sound and true.

Morton laid down guide lines for the prevention of tuberculosis in those deemed likely to develop the disease.

> Therefore, in the preventing of a Consumption, (which is more easier than the Cure of it) the great Business, whilst the Patients remain in this sickly condition, is to take all possible Care that no error be committed in those six things which we call not Natural. For in this so slippery a State of Health, they are wont upon every little Occasion of this Nature to fall headlong into a Fatal Consumption.[15]

His six rules for the avoidance of the 'not natural' were simple and sensible: he advised moderation in eating and drinking, an adequate amount of sleep, moderate exercise daily, the avoidance of strong purges, the laying aside 'care, Melancholy, and all poring of his Thoughts, as much as ever he can, and endeavour to be cheerful' and the enjoyment of 'an open, fresh, kindly Air and such as is free from the Smoak of Coals, which may . . . consequently restore the weak appetite, but likewise procure Quiet (at least in some measure) to the Lungs'.[16] The physicians of later years could not have improved upon this sound advice.

In a subsequent passage when discussing the frequency with which he had observed tubercles in the lungs he added the thought

> Yea, when I consider with myself, how often in one Year there is Cause enough ministered for producing these Swellings, even to those that are

15 Morton, R. (1720) *Phthisiologia.* (2nd ed. Trans) p. 74. London: W. & J. Innys.
16 *Ibid.* p. 75.

wont to observe the strictest Rules of Living, I cannot sufficiently admire that any one, at least after he comes to the Flower of his Youth, can die without a Touch of a Consumption.[17]

With regard to pathology he considered that the tubercles often originated from 'a stuffing of the lung with serum' and held that the changes in the lung were analogous to those noted in scrofulous neck glands, thus echoing the views of Sylvius. He ascribed the fever and other symptoms to a tendency of the tubercles to 'ripen' and turn into cavities. 'For in the Lungs of the dead Body we found at the same time some Tubercles that were turned to Apostemes and others that were inflam'd; and lastly, some that were crude and unripe.'[18]

In his clinical studies he had observed the effect of age on the course of the disease.

> The Consumption of young Men that are in the Flower of their Age, when the Heat of the Blood is yet brisk, and therefore more disposed to a Feverish Fermentation, is for the most part Acute. But in old men, where the natural heat is Decayed, it is more Chronical.[19]

The work of Sylvius and Morton marked an era in the history of tuberculosis for they separated tuberculosis phthisis from other varieties, as well as disposing of the idea that the diagnosis was only permissible in the presence of pulmonary ulceration. They identified the tubercle as a constant specific tissue change, the only specific element which was to be known for the following 200 years, and one which was to become the subject of much theoretical speculation and argument, at times verging upon the acrimonious, among greater and lesser authorities throughout the eighteenth and most of the nineteenth centuries.

Before this argument developed, however, there was a period of relative calm, a sort of academic stalemate, in the early part of the eighteenth century which appears to have been largely the result of reluctance to exchange the comforting shelter of Galenic dogma and infallibility for the pursuit of the new lines of thought which had been opened up. Thomas Sydenham (1624–1689), a contemporary of Morton, despite the great prestige which he enjoyed as a physician made little contribution to the study of phthisis and the chapter 'on coughs and phthisis' in his *Processus Integri* consists only of a brief

17 *Ibid.* p. 88.
18 *Ibid.* p. 102.
19 *Ibid.* p. 121.

description of the symptomatology and some recommendations for treatment. In these he lays particular stress on riding as a sovereign remedy.

> But of all the remedies for phthisis, long and continued journeys on horseback bear the bell; in respect to which it must be noted, that if the patient be past the prime of life, more exercise of the sort in question must be taken than if he were a youth or boy. Bark is no surer a cure for ague, than riding for phthisis.[20]

One of the first to question the teaching of Sylvius, that all tubercles represented glandular changes, was Giovanni Battista Morgagni (1682–1771) who was professor of anatomy at Padua for 56 years and who in his book *De Sedibus et Causis Morborum* practically created the systematic study of gross pathology. He quoted Morton's work, agreeing that phthisis and scrofula were different aspects of the same disease[21] but still believed that there were many different causes for phthisis, the most usual being a certain acrid juice which eroded and ulcerated the lung.

Pierre Desault (1675–1737), a physician of Bordeaux, who for many years had made an intensive study of phthisis and especially of the associated morbid anatomy published a competent dissertation on the subject in 1733. He maintained that tubercles were new structures and not pre-existing glands and he named them as the cause of phthisis, stating that they always preceded haemoptysis. He believed phthisis to be contagious, the contagion being propagated by the sputum,[22] but his views proved unacceptable and lay forgotten and neglected until re-discovered by William Stark nearly 50 years later.

While the glittering stars of the medical heirarchy theorized, argued and made pronouncements, there flashed meteor-like across this firmament of disputation a figure about whom little is known other than his name and the title of his book *A New Theory of Consumptions more especially of a Phthisis or Consumption of the Lungs*. Benjamin Marten (1704–1782) wrote his book in 1719 'from my House in Theobald's Row, near Red Lyon Square in Holbourn' and dated his preface 1 September. He clearly had no illusions regarding the likely fate of his new theory as the opening lines of the preface indicate.

20 Sydenham, T. (1850) *The Works of Thomas Sydenham. II*, Ch. LVIII, p. 296. (Trans. by R. G. Latham) London: Sydenham Society.
21 Webb, G. B. (1) pp. 64–5.
22 Desault, P. (1738) *A Treatise on the Venereal Distemper with Dissertation upon Consumption*. pp. 272–332. (Trans. by J. Andree) London.

There scarcely was ever any Book wrote and published, how good and correct in its kind soever, but what met with Opposition, Censure or Ridicule from People of ill Nature, and of a cavilling Disposition, and that more especially if any Thing New or Uncommon was advanc'd in it . . . that the following sheets therefore, should escape the Splenetic Reflections of insidious Persons, is as far from my Expectation, as their Treatment of them and me, will be from sharing any part of my Concern.[23]

Having done his best to disarm his critics Marten then proceeded with the text of his book, devoting the first section to a general clinical discussion of phthisis beginning with a definition:

a Phthisis or Consumption of the Lungs may be very justly defined to be a wearing away or consuming of all the Muscular or Fleshy Parts of the Body accompanied by a cough, purulent spitting, Hectick Fever, Shortness of Breath, Night Sweats etc.

He continued, referring to the patient's reaction to his afflictions.

Under all which they are supported only by Intervals of Hope that they shall at Last overcome their Distemper and meet with a perfect Cure; which Hope, being the greatest Comfort they have, they very justly endeavour to Keep up in their Minds as much as possible and are fatigued with nothing more than to be discouraged by their Friends and Acquaintances from that the only Enjoyment they seem to have.[24]

A most apt description of the *spes phthisica* which was to figure so regularly among the clinical features of the disease thereafter.

Marten was a strong believer in the contagion of phthisis and in the second section of his book he went on to explain his new theory as to the cause of the disease. He found the theories advanced so far to be unsatisfactory and added that the six 'not naturals' of Morton, although important, could not be the real factors which initiated the illness. 'Yet I cannot help thinking that these are only secondary causes that accidently aid and promote some other Peculiar, Latent or Essential Cause which I suppose must be joined with them.' He then produced his real opinion, the new theory which had prompted him to write the book.

The Original and Essential Cause, then, which some content themselves to call a vicious Disposition of the Juices, Others a Salt Acrimony,

23   Marten, B. (1720) *A New Theory of Consumptions more especially of a Phthisis or Consumption of the Lungs.* pp. 1–11. London: Knaplock.
24   *Ibid.* pp. 3–4.

others a Strange Ferment, others a Malignant Humour (all which seem to me dark and unintelligible) may possibly be some certain Species of *Animalcula* or wonderfully minute living Creatures that, by their peculiar Shape or disagreeable Parts, are inimical to our Natures; but, however, capable of subsisting in our Juices and Vessels.[25]

Later he discussed the probable mechanism of infection.

It may be therefore very likely that by an habitual lying in the same Bed with a consumptive Patient, constantly eating and drinking with him, or by very frequently conversing so nearly as to draw in part of the Breath he emits from the Lungs, a Consumption may be caught by a sound Person . . . I imagine that slightly conversing with consumptive Patients is seldom or never sufficient to catch the Disease, there being but few if any of those minute living creatures . . . communicated in slender conversations, and which, if they are, may not perhaps be produced into Life or be nourished or increased in the new Station they happen to be cast.[26]

Neither Marten's vivid and intelligent writing nor his imaginative but uncannily accurate theorizing struck any responsive chord in the minds of his contemporaries and, unfortunately, experimental medicine had not yet advanced to the point when such a theory was demonstrably capable of scientific proof. His book and his work lay neglected and forgotten (the volume from which these extracts have been taken is one of the very few copies still in existence and is in the possession of the Royal College of Physicians of Edinburgh) but one cannot now deny him the vindication which came his way 150 years later.

During the second half of the eighteenth century fresh impetus was given to the study of the morbid anatomy of tuberculosis by the work of William Stark (1741–1770). A native of Birmingham, of Scottish and Irish ancestry, Stark received his medical education in Glasgow and Edinburgh and on completion of his studies came to London where he obtained an attachment at St. George's Hospital. Here, during the five years of life which remained to him, he made the detailed study of the structural changes in the tuberculous lung for which he is remembered today. He noted that the appearances of the lungs in those dying of phthisis, while uniform, were different in degree and he was the first to examine minutely the growth and

25   *Ibid.* pp. 50–1.
26   *Ibid.* pp. 79–80.

development of the tubercles and to demonstrate how these structures, originally tiny, could lead gradually to advanced disease and death. He wrote thus:

> In the cellular substance of the lungs are found roundish, firm bodies, (named tubercles) of different sizes, from the smallest granule, to about half an inch in diameter; the latter often in clusters. The tubercles of a small size are always solid, even those of a larger size are frequently so; they are of a whitish colour, and of a consistence approaching nearly to the hardness of cartilage; when cut through the surface appears smooth, shining and uniform. No vesicles, cells, or vessels are to be seen in them, even when examined with a microscope, after injecting the pulmonary artery and veins. On the cut surface of some tubercles were observed small holes, as if made by the pricking of a pin; in others were found one or more small cavities, containing a thick white fluid, like pus; at the bottom also of each of these cavities, when emptied, several small holes were frequently to be seen, from which on pressing the tubercle, matter issued; but neither these holes, nor the others above mentioned, (so far at least as could be determined) communicated with any vessels. The cavities, in different tubercles, are of different sizes, from the smallest perceptible, to half an inch, or three quarters of an inch, in diameter; and, when cut through and emptied have the appearance of small white cups, nothing remaining of the substance of the tubercle, except a thin covering or capsule. The cavities of less than half an inch in diameter are always quite shut up; those which are a little larger have, as constantly, a round opening made by a branch of the trachea. At this period, there being a free passage for the matter contained in the tubercle into the trachea, and a communication between the cavity of it and the open air, it is proper to change the name of tubercle to that of vomica.[27]

It is clear from his writings that Stark did not subscribe to the view that the diversity of the pulmonary foci implied that a variety of different diseases was included in the term 'phthisis'. He was describing one disease, and one only, and was proving that the diversity of the structural changes was merely a reflection of local variations in the speed of evolution of the pathological process.

Stark's observations were based on nine cases only, patients who had been under his personal care during life and whose history and symptoms he had recorded in detail together with his postmortem findings. The fact that his work was collected, edited and published after his death suggests that at least one of his colleagues recognized

27 Smyth, J. C. (1788) *The Works of the late William Stark.* p. 26. London: J. Johnson.

the merit of his performance. That same colleague in his preface to the volume gives us a fleeting glimpse of Stark the man.

> Dr Stark was much more conversant with books than with men; possessing great firmness and dignity of mind himself, with uncommon simplicity of manners, he was ill-prepared for the cold prudence; the time-serving meanness, or the base duplicity which he met with in others.

One wonders what lies behind these strong and very revealing words and to what pressures of internal medical politics at St George's William Stark was subjected. One also wonders to what heights he might have risen had not his death at the age of 29 deprived British medicine and St George's Hospital of the services of this brilliant and original research pathologist.

St George's Hospital was to attract another such pathologist within a few years when Matthew Baillie (1761–1823) was appointed to the hospital staff in 1787 at the age of 27. Baillie, son of the professor of divinity at Glasgow and nephew of the Hunters, produced his finest achievement in 1793 with the publication of his *Morbid Anatomy*, the first complete work of its kind. He confirmed the researches of Stark and held that the tubercle was a special formation, starting as a tiny body, no larger than the head of a small pin which grew in the cellular tissue. Adjoining tubercles would coalesce to form larger tubercles. The centre of the tubercle would ultimately change into pus and then go on to abscess formation which Baillie regarded as the cause of phthisis.[28]

Amongst other contributors to the literature of the time was Thomas Beddoes (1754–1808) of Shifnal in Shropshire, who later moved to Bristol where he founded the Pneumatic Institute at Clifton for the treatment of disease by the inhalation of oxygen. In 1799 he published his *Essay on the Causes, Early Signs and Prevention of Pulmonary Consumption* in which he provides some interesting information regarding the incidence of the disease in a non-industrial area. He quotes the parish register kept by the Reverend William Gorsuch of Shrewsbury in which, over a ten-year period, rather more than one death in four was ascribed to phthisis. A similar register from a parish adjacent to Bristol with a population of 10 000 showed that over the seven year period from 1790 to 1796 there had been 1454* deaths of which 683

* In the original text Beddoes gives this figure as 1511, the result of incorrect addition. He was evidently a better physician than mathematician.
28 Baillie, M. (1793) *The Morbid Anatomy of some of the Most Important Parts of the Human Body*. London: J. Johnson & G. Nicoll.

were recorded as being due to consumption or to a 'decline'.[29] These figures are supported by those quoted by Bateman for London where in 1799 he estimated that 1 out of every 3.8 deaths was due to tuberculosis.[30]

Frascatorius had advanced his theory of contagion in 1546 at a moment in history when Italian learning was held in high esteem and in later years support for his views developed particularly in southern Europe where it took an eminently practical form. In July 1699 in the Republic of Lucca the first decree of legislative prophylaxis was promulgated giving the General Sanitary Council of the Republic powers to ensure that

> in future the health of the human body shall not be harmed or imperilled by objects remaining after death of a person suffering from phthisis

and ordering physicians to give notice to the Council of the names of persons treated for or suspected of having the malady. In the middle of the eighteenth century somewhat similar legislation was enacted in Florence when a ban was placed upon the sale of any objects belonging to phthisical patients and those attending upon the sick were warned that

> it shall be the duty of those around the phthisic patient to leave the entrance open from time to time for the egress of fresh air and to take care that he does not empty his sputum except into vessels of glass or glazed earthenware.

In Spain Ferdinand VI introduced compulsory notification of all cases of phthisis and in 1782 Naples also introduced notification requiring in addition that the belongings of a person dying from phthisis should be destroyed unless they were such as to be capable of disinfection. These Neapolitan laws carried heavy penalties for infringement, the edict regarding the destruction of possessions stating

> In the event of any opposition being made the person giving trouble shall have three years in the galleys or in prison if he belongs to the lower class, and three years in the castle and a penalty of three hundred ducats if of the nobility.[31]

It is sad but not surprising that these farsighted and courageous attempts at prophylaxis gradually lost momentum. In Florence the

29 Beddoes, T. (1799) *Essay on the Causes, Early Signs & Prevention of Pulmonary Consumption.* p. 4. London: Longman & Rees.
30 Bateman, T. (1819) *Reports on the Diseases of London.* London.
31 Dubos, R. & Dubos, J. (1953) *The White Plague.* pp. 29–30. London: Gollancz.

law was repealed in 1783, in part because of disagreement among physicians on the question of contagion but also because its enforcement was said to have given rise to 'bitterness, disgust and vexation'. The Spanish and Neapolitan laws, while not fully revoked, gradually fell into disuse, not only because of the expense necessary for their enforcement but also because of the many personal interests involved.

The close of the eighteenth century, therefore, saw tuberculosis raging throughout the land, the failure of early attempts at prophylaxis and a notable absence of any effective method of treatment. While the gross pathology of the disease had been described and its association with the tubercle had been recognized the mode of origin of the latter remained undiscovered. Theories were not lacking, of course, and that enunciated in 1798 by Benjamin Rush (1745–1813) professor of clinical medicine in the Medical School of Philadelphia was a typical sample of the period.

> I yield to the popular mode of expression when I speak of a consumption being produced by tubercles. But I maintain that they are the effects of general debility communicated to the bronchial vessels which cause them to secrete a preternatural quantity of mucus . . . this mucus is frequently secreted into the substance of the lungs where it produces these tumours which we call tubercles.[32]

No agreement had been reached regarding the relationship between tubercles occurring in other areas of the body, particularly in scrofulous neck glands, and those found in the lungs. Indeed most physicians were inclined to look upon these extrapulmonary foci as signs of unrelated diseases. The prevalence of scrofula had led John Coakley Lettsom (1744–1814) to found in 1791 the Royal Sea Bathing Hospital at Margate specially for its treatment[33] yet so little was the disease understood that in 1797 Hufeland in his *Treatise on Scrofulous Disease* wrote:

> If it be true as indeed it cannot be doubted that all the fluids of the human body are specific stimuli that is if they enjoy the faculty of producing impressions that are relative to the sensibility of the vessels which contain them it will doubtless be admitted that this faculty is susceptible of being either augmented or diminished. Now its augmentation is what I call acrimony. In other words whenever any humour is more stimulating than it is in its natural state there is acrimony of that humour.[34]

32 Flick, L. F. (8) p. 319.
33 James, D. G. (1973) Lettsom, Elliot & the Red Barrel. *Hist. of Med.* 5, 21.
34 Flick, L. F. (8) pp. 238–9.

Hufeland goes on to state that the underlying fundamental quality of lymph which makes for scrofula is acrimony, which he terms the scrofulous virus. In addition to the disputes over the pathogenesis of the tubercle and the dreary pages of confused and antiquated theory with which the various protagonists supported their arguments another problem, that of diagnosis, was in need of clarification. So far diagnosis had been based on symptoms and on the patient's general appearance, which meant that the condition was advanced before it was ever considered as a diagnostic possibility. This is borne out by the clinical picture of the consumptive patient which Beddoes described as being characteristic.

> The short teazing cough at first, produced by incessant tickling in the throat, as if the minute fragment of some extraneous body had immoveably fixed itself there; the subsequent hard rending cough, attended sometimes by retching and vomiting, sometimes by stitches which necessitate the most violent struggle against the continued solicitation to cough, and severely punish a moment of inattention; the expectoration sometimes nauseous, always offensive to the eye and harassing when it is not free; the languour with which the patient finds himself overpowered, when his attention is not occupied by some among his various fixed or flying pains; the extremes of cold and heat through which he is carried by the daily returns of hectic; the sweats in which his repose by night drenches him; the breathlessness on motion or without motion, arising by degrees to a sense of drowning, and terminating in actual drowning, when there is no longer strength to bring up the fluids, secreted in the chest; the disorder in the bowels, towards the last always threatening, and finally unrestrainable, while it cuts off those indulgencies which the very thirst it creates or aggravates impatiently demands; – these are but a part of the torments under which the physician, during his transient visit, in an immense majority of instances, sees the consumptive labouring.[35]

But men's minds were now to be applied to the question of diagnosis as, with the close of the eighteenth century, the third period in the history of tuberculosis—the period of physical examination—opens. In this period the scene is switched to Paris where a discovery of lasting benefit to chest medicine was about to be made and where, in addition, the problems of tuberculosis, still disputed in spite of the work of Sylvius, Morton and Stark, were not to be forgotten. These

35 Beddoes, T. (29) pp. 8–9.

were to remain in the foreground and were to command the full attention of those men of genius who were already waiting in the wings as the new century dawned.

Chapter Four
The Period of Physical Examination

The third period in the history of tuberculosis occupies most of the nineteenth century. The opening decades were largely devoted to the exploration of new methods of examining the chest, and these methods stimulated further interest in the pathology of phthisis and in turn, gave rise to a variety of hypotheses and to an argument which raged unremittingly throughout the entire period.

The first tentative steps towards detailed examination of the chest had actually been taken in 1761 when Leopold Auenbrugger (1722–1809) published his *Inventum Novum ex Percussione Thoracis Humani, ut Signo Abstrusos Interni Pectoris Morbos Detegendi*; in this book, destined to become one of the classics of medical literature, he embodied the fruits of his study of percussion. Auenbrugger is said to have started his career with two advantages in that he was the son of an innkeeper and was a good musician, facts which are held to explain much of what was to follow. In his father's inn he had observed the practice of tapping on wine casks to determine whether they were full or empty, but the idea of applying this to the examination of the chest would hardly have occurred to one who had not a good musical ear. A student of van Swieten at Vienna, he later became physician to the Spanish hospital in that city and there began a seven-year study of percussion, experimenting on his patients, checking his findings at postmortems and even introducing water into the thoracic cavities of cadavers so that he might demonstrate the subsequent alteration in the percussion note. In presenting his work he divided it into the following 'observations':

(1) of the natural sound of the chest
(2) of the method of Percussion
(3) of the preternatural or morbid sound of the chest, and its general import

(4) of the diseases in general in which the morbid sound of the chest is observed
(5) of Acute diseases in which the chest yields the morbid sound
(6) of Chronic Diseases in which the preternatural sound is observed
(7) of the preternatural sound of the chest which results from copious extravasation of the fluids contained in the vessels of that cavity
(8) of the affections of the chest which are not indicated by percussion
(9) of the appearances on dissection, in cases where the preternatural sound of the chest has been observed
(10) of scirrhus of the lungs and its symptoms
(11) of Vomicae in general
(12) of Dropsy of the chest
(13) of the Symptoms of a copious extravasation of blood
(14) of Aneurism of the Heart

These indicate clearly the scope and extent of his work. He also remarked in a modest preface:

> In making public my discoveries respecting this matter, I have been actuated neither by an itch for writing nor a fondness for speculation, but by the desire of submitting to my brethren the fruits of seven years' observations and reflexion. In doing so I have not been unconscious of the dangers I must encounter; since it has always been the fate of those who have illustrated or improved the arts and sciences by their discoveries, to be beset by envy, malice, hatred, detraction and calumny.[1]

An even worse fate awaited Auenbrugger for his work was virtually ignored by his colleagues including his old teacher van Swieten. He thus paid the penalty for being ahead of his time and nearly half a century was to elapse before clinical medicine was ready to accept percussion as a valuable diagnostic method.

Recognition came to Auenbrugger ultimately when Jean Nicolas Corvisart (1775–1821), professor of medicine at the College de France and later personal physician to Napoleon Bonaparte discovered his work, hitherto ignored and forgotten, in 1797. Corvisart was that rare animal in eighteenth-century France, a clinician in a country which had as yet no clinical tradition and thus he tended to turn to the Vienna school, the then home of clinical medicine, where he discovered Auenbrugger's treatise and realized that it described a method to approach the examination of the chest of which Paris had

1 Forbes, J. (1824) On percussion of the chest. A translation of Auenbrugger's original treatise. *Bull. Hist. Med. 4*, 373.

never even heard. Determined to put it to the proof, he practised it unceasingly, ultimately delivering his verdict, 'it never led me astray if conditions were such as to allow me to make full use of it'.[2] Apart from adopting the method for his own use he translated and published the original text and when it was suggested that he should write his own book on percussion replied. 'By doing that I would sacrifice Auenbrugger to my own vanity, a thing I shall not do for I wish to revive his splendid discovery'.[3] Backed by the prestige and authority of Corvisart, percussion became widely known and accepted and thereafter retained its place as one of the fundamentals in chest examination.

Corvisart's claims to distinction do not rest solely on his own clinical ability coupled with the acumen which led him to recognize the merit of Auenbrugger's work and arrange for its resurrection. He has another and equal claim to a niche in medical history as the teacher of Laënnec, the greatest of the group of brilliant men who adorned the Golden Age of French Medicine.

To the student of the history of tuberculosis the name of Laënnec will always be associated with that of Bayle. Part of the path which Laënnec was destined to open up had already been trodden by Bayle in making his own contribution to the elucidation of the gross pathology of pulmonary tuberculosis. Gaspard Laurent Bayle (1774–1816) was born at Vernet in Provence and initially was attracted to a career in the Church. Later, feeling that he was unfit for such a calling, he turned to the Law and entered his brother's office. He finally came into medicine almost fortuitously when his political outspokenness during the Revolution made his immediate departure from home imperative. He sought refuge at Montpellier where he entered the medical school and after three years was sent to the Army as a medical officer. While attached to the military hospital at Nice he became interested in pathology and when eventually he reached Paris he strove to perfect his knowledge of both pathology and medicine to such good effect that in 1807 he was appointed to the staff of the Hôpital de la Charité. Three years later he published his most important work *Recherches sur la Phthisie Pulmonaire*, the volume upon which his fame rests. He opened this account of his researches with the declaration that the essential character of phthisis was such that 'Every injury of the lungs,

2 Cummins, S. L. (1949) *Tuberculosis in History*. p. 101. London: Baillière, Tindall & Cox.
3 Beeson, B. B. (1930) Corvisart, his life and works. *Ann. med. Hist. 2,* 300.

which, left to itself, produces a progressive disorganisation of them, and in the end ulceration and death, ought to be called pulmonary Phthisis'. He noted that most physicians appeared

> to have confounded Phthisis with its characteristic signs; and as emaciation and hectic fever are two of the ordinary symptoms of Phthisis, it appears to them absurd to consider that person as affected with Phthisis, in whom they can discover neither fever nor wasting. This manner of considering Phthisis is as ridiculous as that of a naturalist, who having seen a young oak, should refuse absolutely to give it the name, because it does not exhibit as yet all its generic and specific characters . . . So it is with Phthisis: at its commencement it seems hardly a slight indisposition; in its last stages it subdues the stoutest man; . . . Nevertheless it would be unreasonable not to admit that it is still the same disease, and, in order to support the opinion, to rest upon this, that in its first periods it does not exhibit all the symptoms which shall one day characterize it.[4]

These thoughts, the nearest approach to an argument for the earlier diagnosis of phthisis which the literature of the period reveals, prompted Bayle to propose a modification in the current clinical classification of the disease.

> Three stages are admitted in the pulmonary Phthisis, viz.—Phthisis at its commencement, when confirmed, and at the third degree. The commencing Phthisis only takes its date from the origin of the cough, the pectoral oppression, the feverish movements etc; but I think we ought to allow a period before this, when the disease should be designated under the name of occult Phthisis, or the germ of Phthisis; because in many species previous to these symptoms there are intervals during which the patient, who has already the lung deeply injured, appears still to enjoy good health.[5]

But the major portion of the book was concerned with his pathological studies which were extensive and painstaking. He had performed 900 postmortem examinations, many of them on patients whose problems he had already studied at the bedside and on the basis of this formidable experience he wrote:

> Pathological Anatomy compels us to admit six kinds of pulmonary consumption, many of which are sometimes united in the same individual; but they are frequently found distinct, and it is in their simple

4 Bayle, G. L. (1810) *Researches on Pulmonary Phthisis*. pp. 2–5. (English trans. by W. Barrow) Liverpool: W. Grapel.
5 *Ibid.* p. 51.

state that one learns to distinguish them clearly, and at length to discover their complications, whether with one another, or with other diseases.[6]

He later named these six types of phthisis and noted the frequency with which each had been encountered:

Tubercular phthisis	624
Granular phthisis	183
Phthisis with melanosis	72
Ulcerous phthisis	14
Calculous phthisis	4
Cancerous phthisis	3
	———
	900[7]

By so doing he was aware that he was challenging tradition and therefore he set out his reasons.

In the actual state of the Science, it appears to me more suitable to distinguish the species by the different characters of the injury of the lungs, than by the difference of the symptoms alone. Hitherto almost all the physicians occupied with Phthisis have followed a different course in establishing the several kinds of this disorder. They have distinguished them by the symptoms which accompany them – by the causes which determine them or which accelerate their course; and sometimes also by their complications with other diseases . . . This distribution of particular cases of Phthisis, under different titles, is very suitable, especially when writing with practical views; because the species, varieties and even complications which present the same curative indications, are managed under the same title. But in a nosographical sense one cannot admit such species: it is like ranging birds which live on the same nutriment all in one species.[8]

He supported his views by selecting 49 cases for detailed discussion giving, in each instance, a full clinical history followed by a description of the postmortem findings. The clinical and pathological data are both clearly and carefully recorded but he strayed from the path of accuracy when interpreting his observations. Four of his six named varieties of phthisis represented, not separate diseases as he implied, but one disease, tuberculosis, in varying phases of development and in

6 *Ibid.* p. 16.
7 *Ibid.* p. 38.
8 *Ibid.* pp. 17–18.

retrospect it is clear that he had failed to grasp the aetiological identity of one phase with another. Furthermore he had been unable to separate off the cases of bronchiectasis, lung abscess and carcinoma. All this was left for Laënnec to do a few years later but meanwhile Bayle had done a service to scientific medicine by eliminating some earlier misconceptions about phthisis (Bonnafox-Demalet in 1804 had described 12 varieties[9]) even though the fundamental idea of the unity of tuberculosis had eluded him.[10] Whether his industry and interest would have ultimately led him to the truth must remain a matter for speculation for tuberculosis claimed yet another victim in Bayle himself who died from the disease in 1816 at the age of 42.

The work of Auenbrugger and of Bayle in their respective spheres had set the scene for the appearance on the stage of history of one of the greatest clinicians and pathologists of all time, a man who has been justly acclaimed a genius and whose reputation has stood the test of the centuries. René Theophile Hyacinthe Laënnec was born at Quimper in Brittany in 1781. When he was six years old his mother died and, since his father took a light-hearted view of his parental responsibilities, it was considered best that Laënnec and his brother should live with an uncle, the priest of a nearby parish. After one year the boys were transferred to the care of another uncle who was in medical practice at Nantes and it was there that Laënnec entered the medical school in 1795 when he was 14½ years old. His sojourn at Nantes was interrupted by two periods of military service and it must have been with considerable relief that he contemplated the prospect of a move to Paris in 1801. This had become possible when his father was bound by a legal action to supply sufficient money for his board, lodging and fees in Paris where, on 2nd May, he entered the École de Médicine. As well as attending the lectures at the school he attached himself to the clinic at La Charité where he came under the influence of Corvisart whom he admired but did not particularly like. He also became acquainted with Bayle, with whom he was to form a lasting friendship and who was then working hard at morbid anatomy, a pursuit in which Laënnec enthusiastically joined.

A clear and prolific writer, Laënnec was interested in the art of communication and in 1802 he contributed several papers, described

9   Bonnafox-Demalet (1804)*Traité sur la nature et le traitement de la Phthisie Pulmonaire.* Paris: Crappart, Caille et Ravier.
10   Piery, M. & Roshem, J. (1931) *Histoire de la Tuberculose.* p. 249. Paris: Doin et Cie.

as being of 'singular merit', to the journal conducted by Corvisart. In the same year he was awarded the two chief prizes, in medicine and in surgery, offered by the Ministry of the Interior and by 1804 he had acquired such a reputation that he was appointed chief editor of the Journal de Médicine, a post which he held for five years.

During the next decade he developed an interest in diseases of the chest (which he studied intensively both at the bedside and in the postmortem theatre) and in 1816, following the death of his friend Bayle he was appointed physician to the Hôpital Neckar where he began the series of observations which enabled him

> to discover a set of new signs of diseases of the chest, for the most part certain, simple and prominent, and calculated, perhaps to render the diagnosis of the lungs, heart and pleura, as decided and circumstantial as the indications furnished to the surgeon by the introduction of the finger or sound.[11]

In 1819 with the publication of his *Traité de l'Auscultation Médiate* he gave to the world his discovery of the stethoscope. In this first edition he set out the various signs elicited by stethoscopic examination, employing a nomenclature so appropriate that it has remained in use until the present day, followed by notes describing the anatomical lesions with which the signs were associated.

The initial reception of his discovery was cool, as there was a tendency to regard his stethoscope as a mere mechanical toy which had no place in the dignified art of medicine. Forbes, in the preface of his English translation of this first edition, was openly sceptical about its long-term merits.

> That it will ever come into general use notwithstanding its value, I am extremely doubtful; because its beneficial application requires much time and gives a good deal of trouble both to the patient and the practitioner; because its whole hue and character are foreign, and opposed to all our habits and associations. It must be confessed that there is something even ludicrous in the picture of a grave physician proudly listening through a long tube applied to the patient's thorax, as if the disease were a living being that could communicate its condition to the sense without. Besides, there is in this method a sort of bold claim and pretension to certainty and precision in diagnosis, which cannot at first sight but be

11 Laënnec, R. T. H. (1827) *A Treatise on Diseases of the Chest and on Mediate Auscultation.* p. 5. (English trans. by J. Forbes) London: T. & G. Underwood.

somewhat startling to a mind deeply versed in the knowledge and un-
certainties of our art, and to the calm and cautious habits of philosophiz-
ing to which the English physician is accustomed.[12]

Within ten years, however, the doubters and the sceptics had recanted,
auscultation had become established as a most valuable diagnostic
aid, and in conjunction with percussion it remained the only method
available for examination of the chest until the close of the century
brought the discovery of X-rays.

In a second edition of his book, published in 1826, he rearranged
the text so that each disease was described in detail in respect of
pathology, diagnosis and treatment, thus converting the volume into
a complete textbook on diseases of the chest. Of the 393 pages dealing
with diseases of the lungs and pleura 100 are given over to phthisis
pulmonalis, an allocation which is in keeping with the author's own
statement that a quarter to one-fifth of the inhabitants of Paris died
from that disease.[13] Fifty of these pages were concerned with the
pathology of tuberculosis and in these Laënnec proceeded to unravel
much of the tangle in which earlier morbid anatomists had enmeshed
themselves. It is fair to say that Stark and Bayle had glimpsed the
truth which had eluded others but it fell to Laënnec to trace the
evolution of the disease from the tiny grey tubercle onwards through
all its pathological manifestations.

> The matter of tubercles may be developed in the lung, or other organs,
> under two principal forms—that of *insulated bodies* and *interstital injection* or
> *infiltration*. Each of these presents several varieties, chiefly relative to the
> different degrees of development. The insulated tubercles present four
> chief varieties which I shall denominate *miliary*, *crude*, *granular*, and
> *encysted*. The interstital injection of tuberculous matter or tuberculous
> infiltration offers in a like manner three varieties which I term the
> *irregular*, the *grey* and the *yellow*. Whatever be the form under which the
> tuberculous matter is developed, it presents, at first, the appearance of a
> grey semi-transparent substance, which gradually becomes yellow,
> opaque and very dense. Afterwards it softens, and gradually acquires a
> fluidity nearly equal to that of pus: it being then expelled through the
> bronchia, cavities are left, vulgarly known by the name of *ulcers of the
> lungs*, but which I shall designate tuberculous excavations.[14]

12   Dubos, R. & Dubos, J. (1953) *The White Plague*. p. 89. London: Gollancz.
13   Laënnec, R. T. H. (11) p. 311.
14   *Ibid*. p. 222.

It was thus that he declared the unity of tuberculosis, a concept which not even Bayle had envisaged and one that was to be challenged again and again until the arrival of the bacteriological era placed the soundness of Laënnec's observations and deductions beyond all doubt.

He drew attention also to the variations in the lesions noted in different parts of the same lung.

> They begin themselves, in the first place, almost always in the top of the upper lobes, more particularly the right; and it is in these parts more especially that last mentioned that we most commonly meet with the tuberculous excavations of vast size . . . It is more common, however, to find one single excavation and several crude tubercles in a pretty advanced state in the summit of the lungs; and the remainder of these organs, although still crepitous, and in other respects sound, crowded with innumerable tubercles, of the miliary kind, extremely small semi-transparent, and hardly any of them with the yellow speck in the centre. It is evident that these miliary tubercles are productions of a much later date than those which had given rise to the excavations. As well from the result of my own dissections, as from observations of the sick, I am well assured that this secondary crop of tubercles appears about the time when the first set begin to be softened.[15]

It must always be a matter for great regret that Laënnec's untimely death cut short his work on diagnosis before he had had the opportunity to study the earlier stages of the disease. In the beginning quite naturally he concentrated on the advanced cases for it was these which provided the pathological proof of the correctness of his diagnostic findings, but his preoccupation with these grosser manifestations coloured his whole outlook, causing him to write:

> The observations made in the treatise of M. Bayle, as well as the remarks made in the present chapter, on the development of tubercles, sufficiently prove the idea of the cure of consumption in its early stage to be perfectly illusive. Crude tubercles tend essentially to increase in size and to become soft. Nature and art may retard or even arrest their progress, but neither can reverse it. But while I admit the incurability of consumption in the early stages, I am convinced from a great number of facts, that, in some cases, the disease is curable in the latter stages, that is, *after* the softening of the tubercles and the formation of an ulcerous excavation.[16]

15 *Ibid.* pp. 282–3.
16 *Ibid.* pp. 299–300.

Amongst the many services bestowed upon the world by Laënnec should be counted the restoration of hope and confidence to the tuberculous patient which he expressed thus: 'we are still entitled to hope for the cure of many cases of phthisis, or at least, for such a suspension of their symptoms as may be deemed almost equal to a cure'.[17]

Laënnec's exposition of the pathology of tuberculosis, in spite of the convincing detail with which he supported it, gave rise to controversy with another Breton, Broussais. Francis Joseph Victor Broussais (1772–1838) graduated in medicine in 1803, having previously served for a period as a sergeant in the Republican army. He was an army surgeon during the Napoleonic wars becoming principal medical officer in the Peninsular campaign until 1814 when he returned to Paris and was appointed a professor at the Val de Grâce military hospital.

Broussais published his chief work in 1816, producing a volume which caused a considerable sensation at the time since in the course of it he dealt successively, and for the most part unfavourably, with the work of Hippocrates, Galen, Celsus, Paracelsus, Boerhaave, Sydenham and Morgagni; with medicine in Germany, England and Spain; and with contemporary medicine in Paris, where he singled out a number of his colleagues, including Laënnec, for particularly adverse comment. He achieved a reputation considerably in excess of his talents by adopting a simple philosophy of medicine in which he proclaimed that there were no specific diseases and that such entities as cancer, syphilis and tuberculosis were merely the end-result of chronic and often neglected inflammation of the alimentary tract which required only dieting and plentiful bleeding for its treatment. The extreme simplicity of this doctrine and the facility with which it could be introduced into practice made a strong popular appeal and this, added to a vigorous and dictatorial personality, ensured his initial success.[18]

The views of Laënnec ran directly counter to the theories of Broussais, a situation which the latter could not tolerate and a bitter argument ensued which was conducted in the manner customary in that period. Laënnec was no laggard when it came to an exchange of incivilities as the following passage, taken from his second edition and

17 *Ibid.* p. 319.
18 Rolleston, J. D. (1939) F. J. V. Broussais: his life and doctrines. *Proc R. Soc. Med.* *32*, 27.

referring to an utterance by Broussais, indicates. 'More recently this author has impugned the correctness of Bayle's opinion (*Exam. des Doct. Med.* 1816) and he still continues to do so, more by assertion and ratiocination, however, than by facts'.[19]

One cannot record the phenomenal accomplishments of Laënnec during his relatively brief life without commenting on his frail physique and the constant ill-health which afflicted him during his most productive years. A mere 5 feet 3 inches tall, thin almost to the point of emaciation, with prominent cheek bones emphasizing the hollow cheeks, he was the victim of constantly recurring asthma, intestinal complaints and depression, the symptoms of which were at times of sufficient severity as to make continuance of work impossible. At such periods he sought respite in his native Brittany where, with long country walks and shooting expeditions, his health would improve only to relapse again when he plunged back into his working programme in Paris.

In 1823 he had been appointed professor of medicine at the College de France and daily he conducted his rounds at the Hôpital de la Charité where he taught for two hours, mainly in Latin which he held to be the universal language of science as well as an aid to communication with the many foreign students who flocked to his clinic. Around this time he was completing the second edition of his book and it became clear that the effort had taken its toll for his health was now deteriorating. Dyspnoea, cough, anorexia and depression plagued him continuously and when, in May 1825, fever and diarrhoea were added to his ailments it became clear that he was the victim of advanced pulmonary and intestinal tuberculosis. He again sought his home at Kerlouarnec but on this occasion the magic of the Breton air failed him, the deterioration in his condition continued and he died on 13 August 1826, leaving the field of medicine eternally enriched by the fruits of his genius.

Hard on Laënnec's heels came another physician of distinction, Pierre Charles Alexandre Louis (1787–1872). After studying at Rheims, Louis graduated in Paris in 1813. He spent the following six years in Russia until his experiences in a diphtheria epidemic caused him to return to Paris for further education.[20] Here he came initially under the influence of Broussais but, finding cause to query some of

19 Laënnec, R. T. H. (11) p. 290.
20 Steiner, W. R. (1940) Dr Pierre Charles Alexandre Louis. *Ann. med. Hist.* 3rd series, 2, 451.

the latter's pronouncements, decided to turn to research and began an intensive study of tuberculosis. The results of this study, which was based on 123 clinical reports and autopsies on tuberculous patients, were presented to the Royal Academy of Medicine in 1825. His work completely corroborated the findings of Laënnec and confirmed the latter's view on the unity of tuberculosis.[21] He placed the symptoms of the disease in scientific relationship with its pathology; he also divided his cases into two groups, before and after the occurrence of cavitation, and drew attention to the difference in the physical signs. He recognized that pulmonary tuberculosis could exist without producing symptoms and he described extrapulmonary forms of tuberculosis, involving the peritoneum, the larynx and the genital organs, which led him to enunciate the Law of Louis stating that 'after the age of fifteen one could not have tubercles in any organ of the body without at the same time having tubercles in the lung'.[22] Apart from his work, comparatively little that was new was added to the knowledge of tuberculosis by the French School during the 40 years following the death of Laënnec. Outside the exclusive Parisian circle the news percolated through to other European countries and to the United States, exciting comment and provoking argument.

Robert Carswell (1793–1857), professor of pathological anatomy at University College, London, published in 1838 an elegantly illustrated volume, of which the final section was devoted to a discussion of the tubercle. He declared that several eminent pathologists (and it is clear that he numbered himself among the elect) considered that the description of the tubercle given by Laënnec, and later agreed by Louis, was inaccurate since their statement that the grey semi-transparent granulation represented the initial stage of phthisis was erroneous. Carswell then proffered his own opinion:

> The following is, I conceive, a correct definition of tubercle or rather of the tuberculous matter which constitutes the essential anatomical character of those diseases to which the term tubercular is now exclusively restricted. Tuberculous matter is a pale yellow or yellowish-grey, opaque, unorganised substance, the form, consistence and composition of which vary with the nature of the part in which it is formed and the period at which it is examined.[23]

21 Louis, P. C. A. (1925) *Récherches Anatomico-Pathologiques sur la Phthisie*. Paris: Gabon et Cie.
22 Webb, G. B. (1936) *Tuberculosis*. pp. 82–4. New York: P. B. Hoeber.
23 Carswell, R. (1838) *Pathological Anatomy. Illustrations of the Elementary Forms of Disease*. London: Longmans.

Carswell had considerable influence on medical thinking in Britain as had also James Clark (1788–1870) whose *Treatise on Pulmonary Consumption* was probably the best British book on the subject. Clark's text showed that while he was familiar with the work of Stark, Bayle and Laënnec he preferred the teaching of Carswell whose book he described in a fulsome footnote as:

> A work which, whether we regard its beauty and fidelity of execution, or its importance and utility in a pathological point of view, far surpasses any thing of the kind that has been produced in this or any other country.[24]

Although he quoted extensively from Carswell, Clark himself appeared to be somewhat confused on the detailed pathology since he concluded that 'tubercular deposits are always at first fluid, and that the concrete form, in which they are commonly found, arises simply from the absorption of the more fluid part, and is in many situations chiefly dependent on compression'.[25] Clark was also firmly convinced that pulmonary consumption was hereditary and made his attitude clear: 'I regard it as one of the best established points in the etiology of the disease'[26] but he had a sound observation to record when he wrote in his discussion of diagnosis in latent consumption 'Pregnancy appears to retard if not to suspend its progress, and it is frequently observed that it advances with great rapidity immediately after parturition.'[27]

While attention had so far been directed mainly towards the problem of pulmonary phthisis references to non-pulmonary forms of the disease had appeared at intervals in the literature of the times. As far back as 1768 Robert Whytt (1714–1766) of Edinburgh had published a description of tuberculous meningitis and was the first to recognize it as one of the protean manifestations of the disease.[28] Robert Willan (1757–1812), the founder of British dermatology, had written an accurate description of lupus, which he considered to be tuberculous,[29] while Jacques Mathieu Delpech (1777–1832) of Toulouse declared in his *De l'Orthomorphie*, published in 1828, that the spinal curvature and palsy described by Percival Pott in 1779 were caused exclusively by tubercles and should be referred to as 'a tuberculous

24 Clark, J. (1835) *A Treatise on Pulmonary Consumption.* p. 123. London: Sherwood.
25 *Ibid.* p. 258.
26 *Ibid.* p. 221.
27 *Ibid.* p. 57.
28 Comrie, J. D. (1925) An eighteenth century neurologist. *Edinb. med. J. 32*, 755.
29 Willan, R. (1808) *On Cutaneous Diseases.* 1 London: J. Johnson.

affection of the vertebrae'.[30] It was very fitting, therefore, that in 1839 Johann Lukas Schönlein (1793–1864), professor of medicine at Zurich, should suggest that in future the term 'tuberculosis' should be employed as a generic name for all the manifestations of phthisis since the tubercle was the fundamental anatomical basis of the disease.[31]

Another event, relating to the problem of diagnosis, marked the year 1839. This was the publication by Jules Fournet of his work on the early diagnosis of phthisis, in which he called attention to the importance of an increase in the expiratory murmur as a diagnostic sign and endeavoured to give a precise estimate of the degree of difference between the inspiratory and expiratory phases by fixing 10:2 as the ratio of their comparative intensity and duration in the healthy state.[32]

The science of microscopy had now developed to a stage when it could be applied to the study of tuberculosis and its employment soon revived previous doubts and re-opened former arguments. One of the first to study the microscopic structure of the tubercle was Hermann Lebert who in 1845 was awarded the Portal Prize by the National Academy of Medicine in Paris for his essay *A Practical Treatise on Scrofulous and Tuberculous Diseases* which was subsequently published in 1849. Hr regarded tuberculosis and scrofula as separate diseases although they might be associated with one another and occur concomitantly in the same individual while he also claimed to have discovered a microscopic body ('tubercular corpuscle') within the tubercle which he believed to be pathognomonic of the disease and which would serve to differentiate between tuberculosis and other diseases associated with caseation and pus formation.[33]

In 1847 Rudolf Virchow (1821–1902) turned his attention to phthisis and lost no time in the initiation of controversy by declaring that 'tuberculous matter' or caseation was not peculiar to tuberculosis.[34] Thereafter Laënnec's work was heavily attacked. Reinhardt in the *Annals of the Charity Hospital of Berlin* asserted that the tubercle originated with inflammation and that the so-called 'tubercular

30 Webb, G. B. (22) p. 87.
31 Castiglioni, A. (1933) History of Tuberculosis. *Med. Life.* N.S., *40*, 1.
32 Fournet, J. (1841) *Researches on Auscultation of the Respiratory Organs and on the First Stage of Phthisis Pulmonalis.* p. 76. (English trans. by T. Brady) London: Churchill.
33 Lebert, H. (1849) *Traité Pratique des Maladies Scrofuleuses et Tuberculeuses.* Paris: Baillière.
34 Virchow, R. (1847) *Virchow's Arch. path. Anat. Physiol. 1,* 172.

corpuscles' were merely dead and shrunken pus corpuscles derived from ordinary pus.[35] Virchow contributed further to the general confusion by formulating a dualistic theory of phthisis in which he reserved the term 'tubercle' strictly for the miliary granulation and regarded infiltration and caseation, held to be tuberculous by Laënnec, as inflammatory products which he designated caseous pneumonia. The opinion of Virchow that phthisis and tuberculosis were two separate diseases was widely accepted throughout Germany and a leading physician, Felix von Niemeyer, professor of clinical medicine at Tübingen, was constrained to throw overboard the teachings of Laënnec.

> The dangerous tenets of Laënnec's doctrine 'that pulmonary phthisis is a constitutional disease, that it can never develop itself out of acute or chronic pneumonias, or take its rise from a bronchial haemorrhage, or from a neglected or protracted cold' are up to this day taught in the medical schools as undisputed truths and have in practice a most pernicious effect on the prevention and treatment of phthisis. Laënnec's dogma, that every form of pulmonary phthisis is caused by a specific new growth . . . and that the cavities in the lung take their origin alone in the softening and evacuation of this growth, was simply a *pathological hypothesis*, which, by the most recent researches in the field of pathological anatomy, has been entirely refuted.[36]

Niemeyer was wholly convinced by Virchow's declaration that phthisis and tuberculosis were two separate diseases, a view which led him to write that widely quoted sentence from his otherwise forgotten clinical lectures. 'The greatest danger to most phthisical patients is the development of tubercles'.[37] It is hardly surprising that his views on treatment were profoundly influenced by his convictions regarding pathology.

> Against that form of phthisis which consists in a *primary tuberculosis,* as well as against the *tuberculosis which has developed in the course of phthisis*, treatment is indeed impotent and we are simply limited to the palliation of the most troublesome symptoms . . . If we have come to the conviction that a consumptive patient has tubercles, we ought not to send

35   Reinhardt (1850) Uber die Übereinstimmung der Tuberkelablagerungen mit den Entzundungsprodukten. *Charité-Annln* Bd. *I*, 362.
36   von Niemeyer, F. (1870) *Clinical Lectures on Pulmonary Consumption.* p. 1. (English trans. by C. Baeumler) London: New Sydenham Society.
37   *Ibid.* p. 11.

him to Nice, Cairo etc., but ought to let him live his last days among his friends and die in his own house.[38]

Virchow also asserted that phthisis was hereditary and even the observations of Ludwig von Buhl (1816–1880) that miliary tuberculosis was an infectious disease caused by the reception into the blood of the 'tuberculous poison' from pre-existing cheesy foci[39] was lost on him. He was, therefore, ill-prepared to accept the bacteriological area which lay just ahead and which was to obliterate overnight from the tablets of memory much of the dogma and theory of the past.

38   *Ibid.* p. 71.
39   von Buhl, L. (1857) Quoted by von Niemeyer (36) p. 16.

Chapter Five
Bacteriological Proof

The fourth period in the history of tuberculosis lies within the second half of the nineteenth century and is concerned almost entirely with the work of two men. In order to put into proper perspective the magnitude of the contribution which they made to scientific medicine it is necessary to consider briefly the ebb and flow of the argument concerning contagion in phthisis.

Aristotle had held that the breath of the phthisical patient contained something injurious to others which caused them to contract the disease[1] and this view received strong support from Galen who advised against intimate contact with such patients. The Byzantine and Arabian physicians added nothing to the discussion either for or against, while throughout the blank aeons of the Middle Ages the absence of any rigorous isolation such as that imposed upon lepers suggests that phthisis was not then presumed to be contagious. The work of Frascatorius during the sixteenth century re-opened the subject and his views were upheld by many of his contemporaries, one of whom Montano, a physician of Pisa, went so far as to declare that it was possible to develop phthisis by treading with the bare feet on the sputum of a consumptive.[2]

Throughout the seventeenth century the belief in contagion appeared to have found fairly general acceptance save that 'La Faculté de Paris, constamment hostile aux idées nouvelles, se refuse à admettre la contagion'.[3] The eighteenth century saw the enactment of prophylactic legislation in southern Europe but in the north there were signs of diminishing support for the contagionists. William Cullen (1712–1770), the distinguished Edinburgh physician, declared that for

1   Piery, M. & Roshem, J. (1931) *Histoire de la Tuberculose*. pp. 165–6. Paris: Doin et Cie.
2   *Ibid*. p. 169.
3   *Ibid*. p. 169.

phthisis to develop as the result of contagion was quite exceptional, an opinion which he based on his experience with several hundred cases; while Antoine Portal (1742–1832), an equally distinguished French physician with a known interest in phthisis, maintained categorically that the disease was hereditary and had nothing to do with contagion.[4] Bayle believed that heredity was the chief aetiological factor; Laënnec conceded that, although phthisis appeared to be contagious in some countries, this did not seem to be the case in France;[5] while Gabriel Andral (1797–1876), the editor and annotator of the fourth edition of Laënnec's book, although not denying the possibility of contagion, considered that its occurrence was greatly exaggerated.[6]

British physicians appear to have followed the lead given by Cullen. Forbes, in a footnote to his translation of Laënnec's second edition, stated that 'the opinion of the great majority of medical men in this country is opposed to contagion; and I think this opinion is justified equally by statistical facts, by the truths of pathology, and by analogical reasoning'[7] while Sir James Clark, in his *Treatise on Pulmonary Consumption* of 1835, held the view that the disease was rarely acquired by contact and then only by those who were predisposed to it. By the middle of the nineteenth century the contagion controversy had split European medicine into two camps, the southern physicians adhering to their original view and the northerners discrediting the contagion doctrine even to the point where Bricheteau, a physician at the Hôpital Neckar, felt able to write in 1851 'cette conception (la contagiosté) n'a pu naître que dans l'imagination des meridionaux'.[8] It was against this background that Jean Antoine Villemin (1827–1892) stepped forward to begin the series of experiments which were to expose tuberculosis for what it was and to create the run-up to the epoch-making year of 1882.

Villemin, a farmer's son, was born at the village of Prey in the Vosges. He lost his father when he was aged ten and the finance for his studies was provided by an uncle. Originally he intended to be a teacher, but changing his mind during his period of military service, decided to make the Army his career and began studying for the non-

4 *Ibid.* pp. 177–9.
5 Laënnec, R. T. H. (1827) A *Treatise on Diseases of the Chest.* p. 380. (English trans. by J. Forbes) London: T. & G. Underwood.
6 Piery, M. & Roshem, J. (1) p. 182.
7 Laënnec, R. T. H. (5) p. 330.
8 Piery, M. & Roshem, J. (1) p. 183.

commissioned officers' school. His efforts were not successful and on the advice, it is believed, of his colonel, he elected to become an army doctor beginning a course of instruction at the military hospital in November, 1849. He qualified in 1853 and was eventually appointed to the staff of the Val de Grâce military hospital and school of medicine where he became specially attracted by the problem of tuberculosis which seemed to him to have some features in common with glanders, a disease then known to be transmissible by inoculation.

He approached his seniors who eventually found a corner of a laboratory to accommodate him together with the three or four rabbits which were necessary for his research project and in March 1865 he started on the experiments which were to carry him forward to the solution of a great enigma. Using a pair of healthy rabbits he introduced into one, by way of a small subcutaneous wound behind each ear, two small fragments of tuberculous material together with a small quantity of the pus from a lung cavity in a phthisical patient who had died 33 hours earlier. The innoculations were repeated on 30 March and again on 4 April. On 20 June the rabbit was killed and Villemin found tubercles in the peritoneum, along the greater curvature of the stomach and in various other portions of the body 'some showing a little speck in the centre' while the lungs were full of large tuberculous masses[9]. The brother rabbit which had shared everything except the inoculations was also killed and found to be free from disease. He repeated the experiment in six series with exactly similar results. None of the rabbits died from the disease and indeed most of them managed to retain their health throughout the experiment but when Villemin employed tuberculous material from a cow in lieu of a human source the result was strikingly different. The inoculated rabbit rapidly developed signs of severe ill-health and on postmortem examination there was evidence of acute generalized tuberculosis.

The difference was noted by Villemin who commented on the apparent greater severity of the illness in the rabbit when a bovine rather than a human inoculum was used but he failed to draw the vital inference, believing, as all did at that time, that tuberculosis was the same disease whether the host be man or animal. His explanation of his observed phenomenon was that 'This makes one suppose that, like all other virulent substances, tuberculosis acts with the greater

9   Cummins, S. L. (1949) *Tuberculosis in History*. p. 138. London: Baillière Tindall & Cox.

54

intensity when there is a physiological affinity between the creature that furnishes the virus and that receiving it'.[10]

On 5 December 1865 Villemin described his experiments to the Académie de Medicine stating his belief that the results justified the following conclusions (1) tuberculosis is a specific infection, (2) it is caused by an agent which is inoculable, (3) the inoculation from man to rabbit can be readily performed, (4) tuberculosis should therefore be included in the group of virulent diseases, taking its place beside syphilis but closer to glanders. To his bitter disappointment his paper was greeted with a notable lack of enthusiasm amongst the company generally, with the older and more experienced members expressing frank disbelief. To the clinicians, animal experiments in a laboratory could not be related to the clinical problems which they encountered daily nor could transmission by experimental inoculation be considered comparable to the possible pathways of human transmissibility Pidoux, one of the leading physicians of the day, who was about to receive a prize of 10 000 francs from the Faculté de Médecine of Paris for his *Études sur la Phthisie* and who was a firm believer in heredity and a tuberculosis diathesis, would have none of it and the word of Pidoux carried weight. The only acknowledgement to Villemin was a formal and somewhat perfunctory vote of thanks.[11]

Whatever Paris may have thought and felt the work of Villemin did not escape notice elsewhere and in Britain the Privy Council arranged for a visit to France by Dr Burdon Sanderson to collect first-hand information. On his return in conjunction with Dr John Simon of the Local Government Board, Burdon Sanderson proceeded to repeat Villemin's experiments and produced similar results. They took the experiment a step further, however, and inserted setons of unbleached cotton into the shoulders of two guinea pigs. One of these, apart from some local inflammation at the site of the insertion, showed no other tissue changes but the second showed extensive changes in the lungs, liver, spleen and lymph glands which were presumed to be tuberculous. While confirming Villemin's findings, therefore, Burdon Sanderson, in submitting his *Eleventh Report of the Medical Officer of the Privy Council*, added this additional finding with the comment that

the results of tuberculous inoculation could no longer be regarded as necessarily dependent on any property or action possessed by the

10 *Ibid.* p. 139.
11 Piery, M. & Roshem, J. (1) pp. 185–6.

inoculated material in virtue of its having been taken from a tuberculous individual.

This finding suggested a flaw in Burdon Sanderson's technique and additional experiments using similar setons were later carried out, first by Watson Cheyne and subsequently by Dawson Williams, neither of whom succeeded in producing any tuberculous tissue changes.[12]

While the research was in progress one British practitioner, a clinician rather than a pathologist, had become much preoccupied with the problems of tuberculosis. Dr William Budd lived and practised in the city of Bristol, a city which tended to have rather more than its fair share of patients with tuberculosis to whom the milder climate of the south-west had proved an attraction, while its flourishing seaport provided an appreciable number of cases of acute tuberculosis among Negro seamen. Budd had observed the remarkable difference between the chronic disease of the European and the acute fulminating illness which attacked the black seamen and it had puzzled him greatly. In a letter to the *Lancet* dated 1 December 1866 and published in the issue of 12 October 1867 he submitted his thoughts and his conclusions for consideration by others, stating that

> the idea that phthisis is a self-propagated zymotic disease and that all the leading phenomena of its distribution may be explained by supposing that it is disseminated through society by specific germs contained in the tuberculous matter cast off by persons already suffering from the disease, first came into my mind, unbidden, so to speak, while I was walking on the observatory hill at Clifton, in the second week of August, 1856.[13]

He had had, therefore, 11 years to ponder on his original theme and it is clear from his writing that he had thought to good effect, giving weight to what he had observed of the pathology, clinical features and epidemiology of the disease. Had he not been in general practice with its multifarious calls upon his time and energies might he not have taken the course pursued by Villemin and added proof to conjecture? It was not possible for him to do so but he should at least be given credit for the idea and for the astuteness with which he had assessed the facts which he had been able to collect.

Meantime Villemin did not allow his rebuff by the Académie to

---

12 Williams, D. (1884) A preliminary note of some experiments on the etiology of tuberculosis. *Trans. Path. Soc. of London. 35*, 413.
13 Budd, W. (1867) Memorandum on the nature and mode of propagation of phthisis. *Lancet.* p. 451.

deflect him from his path. He pursued his researches and experiments with vigour and tenacity and in 1868 published his results in a book with the title *Études sur la Tuberculose; preuves rationelles et expérimentales de sa spécificité et de son inoculabilité.* In the first 14 chapters he discussed the pathology of tuberculosis, the tuberculous diathesis and the alleged influence of heredity, the physical constitution of the patient and its influence on the disease, occupational factors and the effect of preceding or associated diseases. He was adamant in his belief that tuberculosis was a specific malady and he summed up his arguments in support as follows. (1) Tuberculosis flourishes only exceptionally at high altitudes; (2) it increases proportionately as living conditions become more crowded and is at its maximum in the capitals and in large manufacturing and commercial cities; (3) it afflicts above all individuals who live in common and who are confined indoors; (4) it spares individuals who are scattered, living in the open and in a nomadic or savage state; (5) tuberculosis, so sommon amongst troops in barracks, ceases to be so when the soldier is on campaign and not housed; (6) dwelling together in close badly ventilated houses is followed by tuberculization of many of the occupants; (7) phthisis, unknown among certain people of America and Oceania, became the most violent destructive scourge among them when they came in contact with Europeans; (8) phthisis of the bovine kind, like that of human beings, increases with confinement and crowding of the animals.

In the final chapters he described the experiments which he had carried out to prove his thesis and which included not only the inoculation of tuberculous material from man to a variety of animals but also in turn from animal to animal. For the most the inoculum consisted of material obtained from lung lesions at postmortem but he also used sputum from tuberculous patients and in some cases injected tuberculous material directly into the trachea. He was satisfied that his experiments had proved that tuberculosis was transferable from man to certain kinds of animals and from animals to other animals of the same or different species and that it was, moreover, transmissible not only with the product of the characteristic lesion but also with the bronchial secretions. He finally expressed his conviction that the virus of the disease consisted of a living agent which multiplied and spread in the organism of its host and, speaking in terms of prophylaxis, he advised improvement of housing and working conditions, the maintenance of as high a standard of general health as possible and, where practicable, a return to the practice of disinfecting all things and places which might possibly have been contaminated by consumptives.[14]

Villemin could no longer be ignored and on this occasion the Académie de Médécine appointed a commission to study his work. Their report, apart from a few minor points of disagreement, was favourable but an editorial in the *Lancet* in December 1867 indicated some of the difficulties which the orthodox encountered in accepting Villemin's views. 'To almost disregard hereditary influence, and to be little more respectful of the diathetic peculiarities of the patient, is a bold innovation of teaching on this subject.' Later the writer added:

> While admitting the specificity of the phenomenon resulting in animals from the inoculation of tubercle . . . and impressed with the fact that two observers (M. Villemin and Dr Budd) from different and perfectly independent points of view, have arrived at a zymotic theory of tuberculosis, we cannot but confess the excessive difficulty of reconciling with this theory clinical facts touching the origin and progress of phthisis as we see it in daily experience.[15]

Informed opinion gradually swung in Villemin's favour, some of it admittedly with the maximum of hesitation, but more stout-hearted supporters were to emerge and in 1868 Chauveau reported to the Acadèmie that he had succeeded in producing tuberculosis in three healthy heifers by feeding them tuberculous products.[16] L. Armanni in 1872 inoculated the centre of the cornea of guinea-pigs with a needle dipped in a watery suspension of caseous material and some weeks later watched tubercles develop in the inoculated animals while the controls remained clear.[17] His work, however, was overlooked until, in 1877, Cohnheim and Salomonsen performed a similar experiment, inoculating the anterior chamber of a rabbit's eye and studying the subsequent histogenesis of the tubercles[18] while, also in 1877, H. Tappeiner produced tuberculosis in dogs by spraying their kennels with a dilute solution of tuberculous sputum.[19]

14 Flick, L. F. (1925) *Development of Our Knowledge of Tuberculosis.* pp. 611–42, Philadelphia: published by author.
15 Editorial (21 December 1867) *Lancet* p. 774.
16 Chauveau, A. (1868) De la transmission des maladies virulents par l'ingestion des principes virulents dans les voies digestive. *Gaz. med. de Paris* 47.
17 Brown, L. (1941) *The Story of Clinical Pulmonary Tuberculosis.* p. 24. Baltimore: Williams & Wilkins.
18 Piery, M. & Roshem, J. (1) p. 149.
19 Jaccoud, S. (1885) *The Curability and Treatment of Pulmonary Consumption.* p. 75 (English trans. by M. Lubbock) London: Kegan Paul, Trench & Co.

With the accumulation of such a wealth of evidence one would have thought that the contagion of phthisis could no longer have been denied and yet in the United States in 1881, almost at the eleventh hour, Austin Flint and W. H. Welsh, in the fifth edition of their standard textbook *The Principles and Practice of Medicine*, committed themselves to the statement that 'the doctrine of the contagiousness of the disease . . . has its advocates but general belief is in its non-communicability'.[20]

But the moment of truth had arrived and on this occasion the honour of making a major discovery was to be Germany's in the person of Robert Koch (1843–1910). Koch was born at Clausthal in the Harz mountains. He attended the University of Göttingen, then noted for its Medical Faculty, and graduated with honours in 1866. His immediate postgraduate years appear to have been somewhat unsettled. After a short period of study under Virchow in Berlin he went into private practice in his home town but finding this not to his liking he accepted a hospital appointment in Hamburg. When he had been called up for military service he had been rejected because of defective eyesight but the Franco-Prussian war had since begun and accordingly he presented himself as a volunteer in 1871. He was posted to hospital duties in Orléans and from this post of relative safety, according to the Belgian biographer, Emile Lagrange, he contrived to enjoy his war, finding it 'fraîche et joyeuse'. But all good things come to an end and at the end of the war he settled into an appointment as a District Medical Officer at Wolstein where he gradually developed a taste and a flair for individual research which led him, employing the methods which he was later to make famous, to the discovery of the bacillus of anthrax. An appointment at Breslau followed and a few years later he found himself in a new laboratory in Berlin as an Extraordinary Member of the Imperial Office of Health.

The bacteriological era was now fully launched and as far as tuberculosis was concerned it was no longer a question of *was there a tubercle bacillus?* but rather of who would find it first. Koch threw himself into the search with enthusiasm and determination. Initially his efforts were unsuccessful although the material in which he conducted his search appeared to be that which was most likely to harbour the organisms, namely recently developed grey tubercles taken from the lungs of animals three to four weeks after inoculation. He reviewed

20 Dubos, R. & Dubos, J. (1953) *The White Plague*. p. 69. London: Gollancz.

his technique in search of possible flaws but it was not until he gave further and detailed attention to staining methods that he found the answer. He had noted that in some earlier studies the deepest staining and clearest differentiation of bacteria from surrounding tissues had been obtained when using stains with an alkaline reaction so he decided to employ in his search for the tubercle bacillus an alkaline solution of methylene blue. With this his problem was solved for the rod-like bacilli stood out with startling clarity, especially when Bismarck brown was employed as a background counter-stain.

It was now essential to produce cultures of the organism and after many failures a suitable technique was devised and the series of experiments began which was to prove beyond all doubt that the tubercle bacillus was the cause of tuberculosis. From his previous bacteriological researches Koch had laid down certain postulates which must be fulfilled before a cause and effect relationship could be justifiably established between a germ and a disease. These 'postulates of Koch', which were to become famous, stipulated that (1) the parasite must be found in every lesion in the body (2) it should be cultivated pure, outside the body, for several generations and (3) after pure culture, for sufficient time and for several generations, it should reproduce the original illness in the body of a laboratory animal.

By the beginning of 1882 all was ready and in the cheerless cold and damp of the evening of 24 March the Berlin Physiological Society gathered at 7.0 p.m. in the Reading Room of the Physiological Institute under the chairmanship of Professor du Bois-Reymond. It was a small company, only thirty-six in all, of trained scientists. Amongst them were Helmholtz, Ehrlich and Loeffler but the pathologists, even the great Virchow, were notable absentees as were the leading clinicians.

Apart from an initial somewhat disparaging reference to Villemin's work, believed to have been prompted by considerations of narrow nationalism rather than scientific truth, Koch's paper was a model of what such a communication should be, remarkable alike for its brevity and clarity. After an account of his identification of the tubercle bacillus in every variety of tuberculous product, human and animal, he explained how the bacillus was separated from every other organism and reproduced in pure culture outside the body. This pure culture was then transferred to animals producing in them tuberculous disease, from the lesions of which the bacilli were recovered. The case was complete and irrefutable: tuberculosis, shorn of its mystery, was relegated to the group of infectious diseases while the doctrine of heredity, which for so long had had so many adherents, was shown to be untenable.

It took time, naturally, for this implication of the discovery to sink in, despite the overwhelming evidence produced by Koch. His paper was published in the *Berliner Klinische Wochenschrift* of 10 April 1882 and at the same time he sent a copy to the British scientist, John Tyndall who, realizing the great public importance of the communication, embodied its salient features in a letter to *The Times* newspaper which published it on 22 April. On Sunday 23 April *The New York World* carried a brief cable despatch announcing the discovery and on Wednesday 3 May both *The New York Times* and *The New York Tribune* printed Tyndall's letter in full.

Comments and opinions quickly appeared in the medical journals. At the Annual Meeting of the British Medical Association in Worcester in August 1882 Dr C. Theodore Williams, physician to the Brompton Hospital for Consumption and Diseases of the Chest, addressed the Section of Medicine on the subject of contagion in phthisis. His opening remarks reflect the difficulty which many physicians had in accepting that phthisis was contagious, even in the light of Koch's evidence.

> The chief difficulty lies in the fact that many of the most potent agents of causation of phthisis, such as dampness of soil, bad ventilation, and deficient food, are also conditions which would promote the multiplication of low organisms; and, on the other hand, heredity, which is the source of a large amount of phthisis, cannot be reconciled in its action with the bacillus theory; for, if a man had strongly inherited phthisis in his tissues, are we to believe that the bacilli have been transmitted in the seminal fluid of his father? How can we account for the cases where the parents, having died of consumption, the children are necessarily attacked on arriving at a certain age, with a severe type of the disease? And, moveover, there are several instances—of which one striking one is present to my mind—where the children, who happened to be scattered in various parts of the world, were yet attacked and succumbed to the fell disease at about the same age.[21]

The main text of Williams's paper was based on a study, conducted over a period of 40 years at the Brompton Hospital, where the medical records of all grades of staff, both past and present, were examined

21 Williams, C. T. (1882) The contagion of phthisis. *Br. med. J.* p. 618.

and, when necessary, follow-up inquiries made. This study revealed a very low incidence of tuberculosis among such staff apart from some who developed tuberculosis after leaving the hospital, in which circumstances Dr Williams did not regard their hospital service and their illness as being in any way associated. He concluded that:

1. The evidence of large institutions for the treatment of consumption, such as the Brompton Hospital, directly negatives any idea of consumption being a distinctly infective disease, like a zymotic fever.
2. Phthisis is not, in the ordinary sense of the word, an infectious disease; the opportunities for contagion being most numerous, while the examples of its action are exceedingly rare.
3. In the rare instances of contagion through inhalation, the conditions appear to have been (a) close intimacy with the patient, such as sleeping in the same bed or room; (b) activity of the tubercular process, either in the way of tuberculosis or of excavation; (c) neglect of proper ventilation of the room.
4. In addition to the above, a husband may, though he rarely does so, infect his wife by coition; and this risk is considerably increased in the event of pregnancy.
5. By the adoption of proper hygienic measures, such as good ventilation, and separation of consumptive from healthy people at night, all danger of infection can easily be obviated.

Williams was indeed serving notice that, whatever the laboratories might say, the clinicians would not readily be parted from their profound conviction that heredity was the predominant factor in the aetiology of tuberculosis.

In the United States where 'few of the medical schools of that time made anything more than a pretence of teaching pathology, and bacteriology, then in its infancy, was hardly thought of'[22] adjustment to the discovery and its implications was difficult. Austin Flint, great clinician that he was, immediately on learning of Koch's announcement had sputum examinations carried out on all the patients in his medical wards at Bellevue Hospital. He published the results as an appendix to a re-printing of the fifth edition of his Practice of Medicine, adding his advice that the sputum should be examined in all patients as it would often provide conclusive diagnostic evidence when the symptoms and signs were equivocal. T. M. Prudden of New York, after a series of examinations of sputum and of postmortem

22 Landis, H. R. M. (1932) The reception of Koch's discovery in the United States. *Ann. med. Hist.* p. 531.

material, was enthusiastic about their value, considering that, as a practical measure, the results exceeded what the original report had led him to expect.

There were naturally some dissidents, the most outstanding being Henry F. Formad, a pathologist from Philadelphia. Formad already had an interest in tuberculosis and had formulated ideas about its cause which bore no resemblance to those of Koch. He believed that it was due to an inherited or acquired predisposition, this predisposition consisting of certain tissue differences as compared to the normal or non-predisposed. One year after the discovery Formad was prepared to acknowledge the diagnostic value of finding the bacillus in the sputum but continued to maintain vigorously his disbelief in its aetiological significance and in the contagiousness of tuberculosis. He made his last stand at the meeting of the American Medical Association in Washington in May 1884 where a prolonged discussion took place which has been described as 'the final act in the establishment of the true status of the tubercle bacillus in this country'.[23] Thereafter the diagnostic value of the bacillus and its role as the causative agent of tuberculosis were firmly established, though even then there was no general acceptance of the contagiousness of the disease. The shackles imposed by the deeply ingrained belief in heredity proved difficult to break, leading to delay in the institution of the preventive measures and public health regulations which were so abundantly indicated.

Additional attention was now being directed towards the part played by the bovine bacillus in the pathogenesis of human disease. In his initial writings Koch had given the impression that he considered the human and bovine bacilli to be identical although he did beg leave to reserve final judgment on this point. In 1898 Theobald Smith, working in the laboratory of comparative pathology at Harvard Medical School, showed that the bovine bacillus could be clearly differentiated from the human variety both in its microscopic appearances and cultural characteristics as well as in its toxic properties when injected into a variety of hosts.[24] Subsequently Koch, addressing the Third International Congress on Tuberculosis in London in 1901, indicated his acceptance of Smith's work and of the differences demonstrated between the two varieties but he then went on to express

23 *Ibid.* p. 535.
24 Smith, T. (1898) A comparative study of bovine tubercle bacilli and of tubercle bacilli from sputum. *J. exper. Med. 3,* 451.

his opinion that infection of humans by the bovine organism was extremely rare—so rare, in fact, that the risk from consuming infected milk or beef was virtually negligible. This statement, even though it came from the greatest living authority on the subject, aroused considerable disquiet amongst the audience. Their misgivings were voiced by the President, Lord Lister, in opening the discussion and were echoed by subsequent speakers, who included Bang and Sims Woodhead. So apparent was the public anxiety that, following the Congress, the British Government set up a Royal Commission to study the whole subject. This Commission worked for nine years and its Final Report in 1911 stated that while the human bacillus was the main source of disease in man there could be no doubt that the bovine bacillus was also pathogenic, particularly so in children, although its mortality for all ages was only 6 per cent. Another Commission, set up by the German Government about the same time, had reported in terms which were generally similar.

Thus far the second half of the nineteenth century had proved a period of exciting discovery and of scientific advances in the field of tuberculosis but before the century closed yet another German scientist was to confer further benefits on humanity. On the 23 January 1896, Wilhelm Conrad Röntgen (1845–1923) at a meeting of the Physical Society of the University of Würzburg, announced his discovery of X-rays. This discovery, which was to have far-reaching effects on every branch of medicine, became of special significance in the study of tuberculosis where it was to produce a change in the diagnosis and management of the disease as revolutionary as that brought about by Koch's identification of the causal organism.

The achievements of Koch and Röntgen bring to a close the fourth period in the history of tuberculosis a period which, although brief in time, had seen a marked acceleration in the tempo of discovery. The results of these crowded years were to produce their full effects in the twentieth century when man, no longer fighting the unknown, but an enemy named and visible, went over to the offensive. The offensive burgeoned into an all-out campaign, a war fought on the two fronts of treatment and prevention, and it is the story of this war, with its swings of fortune followed by ultimate achievement, which forms part two of the history of tuberculosis.

Chapter Six
Treatment from the Renaissance until Koch

The unmasking of *Mycobacterium tuberculosis* by Robert Koch added a stimulus, hitherto lacking, to the search for an effective treatment for the disease. Koch himself bent his energies and intellect to the project but, before telling of his contribution and of its outcome, a review of the therapeutic scene from the Renaissance up to November 1882, may be helpful by providing the backcloth against which the struggle with tuberculosis, about to enter a new and dramatic phase, can be portrayed.

The original hygienic/dietetic regimen of Hippocrates and Galen, as laid down in the translations of the great Greek texts, continued to form the basis of treatment by the Renaissance physicians in conjunction with the medicaments favoured by Galen. Practice changed little in the seventeenth century except that exercise, particularly horse-riding, came into favour—largely as the result of Sydenham's enthusiasm. It is possible, however, in this period to detect a note of dissatisfaction with the customary medication creeping in, a dissatisfaction which found expression in the prompt employment in the treatment of phthisis of every new substance imported into Europe. Quinine, tea, coffee, cocoa and even tobacco all had their vogue and their adherents. There were also some who believed that local applications, usually reserved for cases of scrofula or rheumatism, would be equally efficacious for phthisis and of these preparations human fat was the most highly prized. It was stocked by all apothecaries who, obtaining their supplies from the executioners, produced an acceptable end-product by compounding it with aromatic herbs.[1]

Towards the latter part of the eighteenth century there appeared a tendency to advise residence in the country, combined with moderate

1 Piery, M. & Roshem, J. (1931) *Histoire de la Tuberculose.* pp. 165–6. Paris: Doin et Cie.

riding or light work in the fields or garden, while spa treatment also became popular, especially in France. Detailed attention was given to diet which, it was considered, should be moderate in quantity and consist of easily digested foods, with the French physicians in general disapproving of their British colleagues habit of permitting a generous intake of beef and alcohol.

It is clear from the literature of this period that some of the leading clinicans were now attempting to adjust their treatment of phthisis to conform with their assessment of the stage of the disease. Thus in the initial 'inflammatory' phase, the stage of plethora, an 'antiphlogistic' regimen of blistering, vomiting, purging, bleeding and a light diet was indicated while in the second phase, that of 'ulceration', balsams, expectorants, lime water and opium constituted the main therapy.

The opening years of the nineteenth century were therapeutically disastrous due to over-enthusiasm, which was sustained and nourished by the simple 'irritation' doctrine of Broussais, for 'antiphlogistic' therapy and bleeding. The cautery and the blister came into ever-increasing use while blood flowed in torrents. Broussais set forth his indications for venesection quite simply.

> With a strong pulse and a strong patient, I bleed. With a strong pulse and a weak patient, I bleed. With a strong patient and a weak pulse, I prefer to bleed. With weakness of both patient and pulse bleeding is contra-indicated.[2]

This therapeutic exsanguination was accompanied by a diet which was light to the point of absurdity since it consisted of approximately two pints of milk with two to four ounces of bread daily.

The poet John Keats fell victim to the practices of the period and his story makes sorry reading. Already suffering from an undiagnosed phthisis he had a sudden haemoptysis on returning to his Hampstead Heath home one cold winter's night. A surgeon was called and the customary bleeding was carried out to such effect that at 5.0 a.m. the patient fell asleep from sheer exhaustion. Thereafter he was seen by a series of medical advisers including one, Robert Bree, a Fellow of the Royal College of Physicians, who for a time took charge of the case. Bree's reputation rested largely on his claim to be able to cure asthma by the prescription of digitalis and he felt that there was nothing to be lost by trying this remedy in the poet's case. Digitalis was thereupon

2 *Ibid.* p. 369.

administered in doses large enough to produce nausea while, to add to his miseries, a very light and entirely meat-free diet was prescribed. At no stage was there any suggestion that the patient be advised to rest.

The progression of the disease with its accompanying fever, recurrent haemoptysis, lassitude and depression led his advisers to suggest that he spend the winter of 1820 in Italy which he reached after a stormy and protracted voyage during which he was much afflicted by seasickness. Installed in lodgings in Rome he came under the care of Dr James Clark, later Sir James, who was then practising in Italy and from whom he received great kindness and attention. Unfortunately Clark's medical management of the case was as uninspired as that of his predecessors. After seeing Keats for the first time he even appears to have been in a quandary over the diagnosis in spite of the lassitude, the emaciation, the fever, the cough and the frequent episodes of haemoptysis, since he wrote to a medical friend about the case: 'The chief part of his disease seems to be in his stomach. I have some suspicion of disease of the heart, and it may be of the lungs, but say nothing of this to his friends'.[3] The glaring truth ultimately became obvious even to Clark but this revelation brought no relief to the stricken poet. The scanty diet was continued and each recurrence of haemoptysis was the signal for yet further venesection. Thus assisted by the therapy of the times, the patient's condition deteriorated steadily until he died in February 1821 five months after his arrival in the Italy from which he had hoped to gain so much.

It is fair to say that Laënnec never lent his authority to these rigorous regimens. He expressed his views on bleeding quite briefly.

> Bleeding can neither prevent the formation of tubercles nor cure them when formed. It ought never to be employed in the treatment of consumption except to remove inflammation or active determinations of blood, with which the disease may be complicated.[4]

He was a strong believer in climatotherapy and particularly in the benefits of sea air, a belief which led him to strew seaweed, transported from Brittany, around his wards in Paris thus evoking a torrent of sarcasm from the Broussais camp. Apart from his moderation in the

3 Pitfield, R. D. (1930) John Keats: The reactions of a genius to tuberculosis and other adversities. *Ann. med. Hist.* 2, 530.
4 Laënnec, R. T. H. (1827) *A Treatise on Diseases of the Chest.* p. 362. (English trans. by J. Forbes) London: T. & G. Underwood.

use of venesection and his predilection for seaside air, his treatment was directed largely towards symptomatic relief.

> If we are destitute of every direct and effectual means of resisting this disease we are, at least, able in many cases to alleviate its most troublesome symptoms such as the cough, dyspnoea, night sweats and diarrhoea.[5]

The conspicuous lack of success attending 'antiphlogistic' therapy and bleeding inevitably led some to question the wisdom of such a programme. One notable rebel against the orthodoxy of the period was Dr George Bodington of Sutton Coldfield who in 1840 published his *Essay on the Treatment and Cure of Pulmonary Consumption.* In this he attacked vehemently

> the helpless and meagre system of medical treatment of consumption in general use at the present day, the utter uselessness of which is so well-known and so obvious, that the members of the medical profession in the towns are in the habit of dismissing their patients to some distant sea-port or watering-place, where, falling under precisely the same mode of treatment, they there commonly die.

He condemned the use of the two popular drugs of the day, digitalis and tartar emetic, as well as the practice of shutting patients up in a close room from which fresh air was as far as possible excluded. He proposed a vastly different regimen based upon

> the most important remedial agent in the cure of consumption, that of the free use of a pure atmosphere; not the impure air of a close room, or even that of the house generally, but the air out of doors, early in the morning, either by riding or walking; the latter when the patients are able, but generally they are unable to continue sufficiently long in the open air on foot, therefore riding or carriage exercise should be employed for several hours daily, with intervals of walking as much as the strength will allow of, gradually increasing the length of the walk until it can be maintained easily several hours every day . . . The patient ought never to be deterred by the state of the weather from exercise in the open air; if wet or rainy, a covered vehicle should be employed, with open windows. The cold is never too severe for the consumptive patient in this climate; the cooler the air which passes into the lungs, the greater will be the benefit the patient will derive. Sharp frosty days in the winter season are most favourable. The application of cold pure air to the interior

5   *Ibid.* p. 320.

surface of the lungs is the most powerful sedative that can be applied, and does more to promote the healing and closing of cavities and ulcers of the lungs than any other means that can be employed.[6]

Bodington took a house at Maney close to his own home for

the reception of patients of this class who may be desirous, or who are recommended to remove from their homes for the benefit of change of air etc. It is presumed that, as the situation is very superior in point of dryness, mildness, and purity of air, the advantages to be derived from systematic arrangements with regard to exercise, diet, and general treatment, with the watchfulness daily, nay, almost hourly, over the patient of a medical superintendent, great advantages may be obtained by the consumptive patient treated in this way, in comparison with those to be obtained by the removal of such a one to a boarding home or hotel merely for change of scene.[7]

In addition to fresh air he allowed his patients 'a nutritious diet of mild, fresh animal and farinaceous food, aided by the stimulus of a proper quantity of wine, having regard to the general state and condition of the patient'. He made little use of drugs other than for sedation and for this purpose he preferred morphine, giving a 'full dose of the hydrochlorate' at night with smaller doses two or three times during the day.

Bodington's humane and innocuous regimen was bound to prove superior to the bleeding, blistering, purgation and starvation which was the recognized treatment of the day and he cites in his essay a series of five successfully treated cases. Two of these may have been cases of lung abscess but the remaining three bear the hall-mark of pulmonary tuberculosis and the patients made good recoveries.

When one considers the usual fate of the patient with tuberculosis at that period one might have expected some favourable, albeit cautious, comment on Bodington's work and a sufficiency of interest to encourage others either to confirm or refute his thesis by clinical trial. Instead the medical establishment closed ranks and a review in the *Lancet* in July 1840 administered the *coup de grâce*.

The modest and rational preface with which the author introduced to us his pamphlet on pulmonary consumption, has so far influenced us, that we shall merely give an outline of his principles, without expending

6 Bodington, G. (1840) *An Essay on the Treatment and Cure of Pulmonary Consumption.* pp. 16–17. (Reprinted 1906) London: Simpkin, Marshall, Hamilton & Kent.
7 *Ibid.* p. viii.

any portion of our critical wrath on his very crude ideas and unsupported assertions.[8]

Disheartened by the reception of his ideas and methods, Bodington relinquished his interest in tuberculosis though he still continued in general practice in Sutton Coldfield.

The *Lancet* reserved its *amende honorable* for his obituary notice in its issue of March 11 1882 when, after outlining his career, the reviewer went on to speak of his essay on *The Treatment and Cure of Pulmonary Consumption*.

> In his little book Dr Bodington anticipated by many years the modern view of the treatment of phthisis . . . It is remarkable that a village doctor should have arrived in 1840 at these conclusions, which anticipated some of our most recent teachings. It is less remarkable that he met with the usual fate of those who question authority. He was severely handled by the reviewers, and so discouraged from pursuing observations which might have been of the greatest value. In 1857, some years after he had given up general practice, a writer in the *Journal of Public Health* unearthed Doctor Bodington's treatise, and did him tardy but ample justice. We are glad again to claim for a general practitioner the high credit of having been the first, or among the first, to advocate the rational and scientific treatment of pulmonary consumption.[9]

It can fairly be asserted that George Bodington was the progenitor and pioneer of the sanatorium treatment which in future years was to constitute the main line of defence against the disease. The credit for the introduction of this treatment is usually given to Brehmer and Dettweiler but it would be an act of gross injustice if one did not pause to spare a thought for the Warwickshire practitioner whose humanity and common sense allowed him to see and to assess at their true value the excesses which, in the name of therapy, were being perpetrated daily by his seniors and his contemporaries.

The revolt against the 'antiphlogistic' school of therapeutics continued and in 1853 John Hughes Bennett, professor of clinical medicine at Edinburgh, was writing concerning this treatment.

> It consisted of antimonials, cough mixtures and opiates, leeches applied frequently to the chest and occasionally general bleeding; sulphuric acid to relieve the sweating; astringents to stop diarrhoea or haemoptysis; now and then counter-irritants and towards the termination of the

8 Review of Mr Bodington on Consumption. (July 1840) *Lancet*, 575.
9 Obituary: George Bodington M. D. (March 1882) *Lancet*, 417.

disease, wine and stimulants. As diet, milk and farinaceous foods were the rule and meat the exception. Under such a system of practice, it need not be wondered that consumption should be regarded as almost a uniformly fatal disorder.[10]

Having delivered this broadside Bennett had to suggest an alternative and he unhesitatingly selected cod-liver oil, for which he claimed specific curative properties in the treatment of phthisis. He based his claim on his belief that

pulmonary tuberculosis is a disease of the primary digestion causing—1st, impoverishment of the blood; 2d. Exudations into the lung, which present the characters of tubercular exudation; and 3d. Owing to the successive formation and softening of these, and the ulcerations which follow in the pulmonary or other tissues, the destructive results which distinguish them.[11]

He developed his theme by selecting as his first objective the improvement 'of the Faulty Nutrition, which is the cause of the Exudation assuming a Tubercular Character' and in order to achieve this improvement he believed that a considerable increase of fat in the diet was essential. This fat he supplied in the form of cod-liver oil in a dose of one to six tablespoonfuls daily. He found this treatment to be well tolerated but occasionally encountered 'a few rare cases' in which the digestive system rejected the oil. To cope with this situation he arranged with a firm of apothecaries in Leith Walk to provide him with a cod-liver oil ointment but unfortunately the patients found the constant smell of the oil to be even more disagreeable than the unpleasant taste and eructations. As a last resort, and on the suggestion of a Dr Buist of Aberdeen, he tried a oleaginous enema consisting of 'two wine-glassfuls of cod-liver oil, a table-spoonful of wine, the same quantity of arrowroot, beat up with eight or ten ounces of warm water, to which was added sixty drops of laudanum.' He admitted to some temporary success in a few cases but feared that 'the objection to the constant use of enemata will, by the majority of persons in this country, be stronger than that against continued inunction.' It is said that his enthusiastic advocacy of cod-liver oil increased its sale by one Edinburgh business house from 1 gallon to 600 gallons a year![12]

10 Bennett, J. H. (1853) *The Pathology and Treatment of Pulmonary Tuberculosis.* p. 82. Edinburgh: Sutherland & Knox.
11 *Ibid.* p. 60.
12 Webb, G. B. (1936) *Tuberculosis.* pp. 150–1. New York: P. B. Hoeber.

Apart from his obsession with cod-liver oil his treatment appears to have been reasonable. He was strongly averse to bleeding, used blisters sparingly and deprecated the practice of sending confirmed phthisical patients abroad in search of health. He believed exercise to be beneficial, whether taken on foot or on horseback, provided that the patient was sheltered from cold winds, and foresaw how certain advantages might accrue to the tubercular from the new Crystal Palace at Sydenham to which they could be transported by a closed carriage in the worst weather and, once inside the building, 'could breathe for hours a pure, balmy air, meet their friends, take exercise in various ways, read, work or otherwise amuse themselves.'

Meanwhile the public conscience had been stirring uneasily in contemplation of the problem which had been created by tuberculosis and the inadequacy of the measures available for its solution. By 1840 England had a population of 15 millions, of which one-eighth were crowded into London, and an annual tally of nearly 60 000 deaths from tuberculosis. The combination of disease and child labour had reduced the life expectancy of a working man to little more than 17 years. Publications such as Engel's *The Condition of the Working Class in England* had endeavoured to focus attention on this deplorable situation but even more effective as propaganda were the novels of Dickens and Kingsley which struck home to a wider public.

The forces of humanitarianism began to gather and one of the first manifestations of the new spirit was the foundation in 1841 of the Brompton Hospital for Consumption and Diseases of the Chest. The small incident which led to the birth of this famous hospital began when a city clerk, who was suffering from tuberculosis, failed to gain admission to a general hospital. He had been held in high regard by his employer who took the initial step towards preventing the recurrence of such a situation by organizing a public meeting 'to consider the founding of a hospital as an asylum for consumptive patients and as a means of furthering knowledge of the disease'. As a result of this meeting temporary premises were leased to provide accommodation for 20 patients while plans were prepared for the building of a new hospital on a site which had been acquired at Brompton, a village of Kensington 'remarkable for the salubrity of its air'.[13] The foundation stone of the new hospital was laid on 11 June 1844 by the Prince Consort and the first 60 beds were in use by November

13   Hoyle, C. (1948) The Brompton Hospital: A centenary review. *Dis. Chest, 14*, 269.

1846. The City of London Hospital for Diseases of the Chest in Victoria Park followed in 1851 and by 1886 there were 19 hospitals for tuberculosis in England and Wales.[14]

It would have been pleasant to record that this action by an enlightened and progressive public produced an immediate dividend in the form of improved methods of treatment but unfortunately there is no evidence that such was the case. In 1858 Dr Robert Payne Cotton, physician to the Brompton Hospital, published his book *On Consumption* in which his treatment followed closely that recommended by Hughes Bennett and thus was at least relatively harmless[15] but in 1865 Dr James Edward Pollock, also a physician to the Brompton Hospital, wrote on *The Elements of Prognosis in Consumption*. The portion of this book which deals with the natural history of tuberculosis is excellent and in advance of the period but unfortunately the author was tempted into incorporating a section on treatment in which he advocated methods remarkably similar to those which Bodington had castigated 18 years earlier. He considered that, from the moment that one could detect by physical examination the existence of deposit in the lung, which he held to be the result of congestion, a policy of local depletion was indicated

> as the necessary, if not the sole, mode of relief in the early days of a declared deposit in the lung with irritative fever. The common case of a florid haemoptysis, with high pulse, a daily febrile access and sweating, where dullness and feeble respiration, with prolonged expiration, are ascertained to exist at one apex, ought to be actively treated by local depletion, followed by counter-irritation. A few leeches, followed by the cupping glass over the seat of dullness, saline medicines, perfect repose and a non-stimulant diet, offer the best chances of ensuring quiescence of the deposit which has already taken place.[16]

Later when dealing with the treatment of chronic cavitation he writes:

> It is in this case that counter-irritation is of such a marked use, and the best of all modes is the seton. When the cavity has been fully formed and remains stationary in its limits, as evidenced by the physical signs beneath

14 Meachen, G. N. (1936) *A Short History of Tuberculosis.* p. 19. London: J. Bale, Sons & Danielsson.
15 Cotton, R. P. (1958) *On Consumption: its Nature, Symptoms and Treatment.* pp. 185–290. London: J. & A. Churchill.
16 Pollock, J. E. (1865) *The Elements of Prognosis in Consumption.* p. 399. London: Longmans, Green & Co.

it, and when flattening of the chest wall is beginning to take place, a seton should be placed over the spot. If this be objected to, an issue or perpetual blister is to be maintained.[17]

Britain did not drift alone in these therapeutic doldrums. The golden age of French medicine appeared to have lost its radiance and evidence for this can be found in the writing of S. Jaccoud who in 1881 published his book *The Curability and Treatment of Pulmonary Phthisis*. Jaccoud, professor of medical pathology to the Faculty of Paris, a member of the Academy of Medicine, and physician to the Lariboisière hospital, is said by his English translator to be 'generally recognized on the continent as one of the best authorities on pulmonary phthisis' and in his book he devoted 336 of its 397 pages to treatment. He wrote enthusiastically and at length of an extensive variety of medicaments, to the use of which he ascribed 'some of the most brilliant successes of my practice'. He believed whole-heartedly in the benefits of counter-irritation for every form of pyrexia, whether congestive or inflammatory, provided that such counter-irritation was perseveringly employed and instructed as follows:

Of the different modes of practising counter-irritation already considered, the successive application of blisters seems preferable to the others. In many cases it may be useful to provoke and maintain suppuration at the surface—a practice undoubtedly painful; but when the local lesions are recent, large in size, stationary, and threaten to remain in the acute condition, such treatment is more beneficial than counter-irritation of a less energetic or prolonged character. Upon this subject I again speak from experience and cannot sanction the discredit into which this mode of treatment has fallen, no absolute counter-indication existing to its use except intense constitutional debility.[18]

He devoted an entire chapter to treatment by mineral waters and no less than three chapters to climatic treatment. The value of his methods as a serious contribution to medicine may, perhaps be best assessed by a study of his recommendations regarding milk.

If possible, the milk should be drunk in the cowshed at the time of being drawn, and it is only when the repugnance to this method cannot be overcome that it should be taken cold. In addition to its favourable action upon the digestive functions and secretions of the kidneys, milk taken

17 *Ibid.* p. 408.
18 Jaccoud, S. (1855) *The Curability and Treatment of Pulmonary Phthisis*. p. 190. (English trans. by M. Lubbock) London: Kegan Paul, Trench & Co.

in this way has the great advantage of diminishing the frequence and intensity of the cough, and after a time has undoubtedly a sedative effect upon nervous or vascular excitability. Frequently repeated observations enable me to make this statement with certainty, and such effects are more rapidly produced and more decided when the patient is accustomed to take milk in the cowshed itself and to remain there for some minutes . . . Breathing this air during a length of time which varies from three quarters of an hour to an hour daily, and divided into four or five different periods, is perfectly compatible with other therapeutic requirements, and as I am convinced of the advantages of this practice I recommend it without hesitation . . . my conviction is so strong that I give this advice even to patients who are unwilling or unable to take milk. Such cases undoubtedly exist, though they are uncommon; and in making this recommendation, I at any rate feel sure that, while losing the complex advantage derived from the milk, I obtain the calming effect which this atmosphere has upon the cough and bronchial irritation.[19]

Later, in discussing climatic treatment of phthisis and its associated requirements, he emphasized that 'any place aspiring to the treatment of phthisis shall afford means of treatment by the milk of the cow, goat or ass taken in the shed'.[20]

In this therapeutic desert of the nineteenth century there was but one oasis, and that in Germany, where a project was conceived and developed which was to have far-ranging repercussions for the treatment of tuberculosis over the next 100 years. The story of this project centres on one man, Hermann Brehmer, who was born at Kurtsch in Silesia on the 4 August, 1826. He studied at the universities of Breslau and Berlin taking natural philosophy and mathematics; but, attracted by the work of the great physiologist, Johannes Muller, he forsook mathematics for medicine. After graduation he began to practice in the small village of Gorbersdorf which at that time had no more than 900 inhabitants. Brehmer had already decided on his life's work for he had chosen as the subject of his final graduation address *De Legibus ad initium atque progessum tuberculosis pulmonum spectantibus* (The laws concerning the beginning and progress of tuberculosis of the lungs) electing to defend the thesis that 'Tuberculosis of the lungs in the beginning is always curable.'[21] He had formed certain views on the cause of tuberculosis, based on

19 *Ibid.* pp. 127–8.
20 *Ibid.* p. 330.
21 Brown, L. (1941) *Story of Clinical Pulmonary Tuberculosis.* p. 94. Baltimore: Williams & Wilkins.

75

observations which he had made during his pathological studies, when he had noted an apparent disproportion in the relative size of the heart and lungs in patients dying from phthisis. The lungs appeared large while the heart was small with thin, relaxed and weakened muscular walls. From this Brehmer argued that the small weak heart must result in a diminished circulation, leading consequently to an insufficient pulmonary blood supply and to poor general nutrition. This, he believed, could be offset by residence at an altitude well above sea-level where the reduced atmospheric pressures could produce an increase in heart action followed in turn by an increased metabolism. He linked his theory to the alleged relative immunity to phthisis of the inhabitants of mountainous areas which had been noted by Hufeland and Schonlein and which Lombard of Geneva claimed to have confirmed by researches in the Swiss Alps.[22] In addition to altitude his other requirements for treatment included an abundant supply of rich food, some alcohol, hydrotherapy and regular physical exercise under constant medical supervision—all with the aim of strengthening the heart and improving the pulmonary and general circulation and the nutrition.

Having formulated his plan of treatment Brehmer now faced the problem of putting it into practice. Suitable premises had to be built and for this government permission was required. The Prussian government showed no disposition to co-operate due, it is believed, to Brehmer's well-known and highly democratic ideas, which were not of a nature likely to earn the commendation of higher authority. Fortunately he had equipped himself with the first essential in dealing with intransigent government departments, namely influential friends, and, thanks to the intervention of Johan Lukas Schonlein and Alexander von Humboldt, permission to build was eventually forthcoming. Thus in 1854 the first sanatorium built exclusively for the treatment of pulmonary tuberculosis came into being.[23]

It is probably unnecessary to record that Brehmer did not immediately achieve international fame as the pioneer of a great new conception. The first edition of his book *Chronic Pulmonary Consumption and Tuberculosis of the Lung* was published in 1857 and attracted only one review and that unfavourable.[24] A second edition in 1869 was accorded a better reception and as his methods and results

22 Piery, M. & Roshem, J. (1) pp. 385-7.
23 Knopf, S. A. (1904) Hermann Brehmer. *N.Y. St. med. J., 80*, 1.
24 Brown, L. (21) p. 95.

became more widely known the sanatorium at Gorbersdorf took on a new dimension, becoming the prototype for those others which were to follow in Europe, in the United States and eventually in every civilized country in the world.

Those who knew Brehmer have described him as a striking personality, imposing in appearance and with boundless energy. His patients had implicit confidence in him although a few of his contemporaries accused him both of undue brusqueness and imposing an over-severe discipline. He could certainly be forthright and amongst the *obiter dicta* attributed to him is the statement that the two great causes of death in tuberculosis had little to do with the disease itself but were due to lack of discipline on the part of the patient and to carelessness on the part of his doctor,[25] an utterance hardly calculated to win him friends amongst his own profession. It fell to Flugge to say the final word when in an obituary he wrote 'People, always charming and polite, have never yet accomplished such titanic labors as are represented in the life of Brehmer'.[26]

Although the reasoning behind Brehmer's scheme of treatment was fallacious his results were better than those obtained by the orthodox methods of the day, a fact which need occasion no surprise. The next step forward was to be taken by Peter Dettweiler, who, having been a patient of Brehmer's, was thereafter his assistant until he left to found his own sanatorium at Falkenstein in the Taurus mountains in 1876. Dettweiler was not particularly impressed with the role of altitude in treatment but he was most firmly convinced of the great therapeutic advantages of fresh air while he also believed that rest should play a more dominant part in treatment than that assigned to it by Brehmer. In order to combine the maximum amount of rest with the maximum amount of fresh air he erected pavilions near the entrance to the sanatorium where the patients either in their beds or, suitably wrapped up, in *chaises longues* could spend many hours in the fresh air. 'In spite of rain, fog, winds and snow, in spite of a temperature often below 12°, very often without sun, the patients had their daily treatment of seven to ten hours, sometimes even twelve'.[27] Unlike Brehmer he had considerable reservations about exercise which, for many patients, he regarded as unwise and only to be prescribed with great caution. Diet figured prominently in the Falkenstein programme, the

25 Piery, M. & Roshem, J. (1) p. 386.
26 Knopf, S. A. (1904) Hermann Brehmer. *N.Y. St. med. J.*, *80*, 1.
27 Piery, M. & Roshem, J. (1) p. 389.

patients having six meals daily of food rich in fats and carbohydrates, while medicines were kept to a minimum since Dettweiler held the enlightened view that, as far as tuberculosis was concerned, all medicines were non-specific and frequently useless. He would use them only when indicated for the relief of symptoms and he considered alcohol, given as wine or cognac, to be one of the few true medicaments.

The ideas of Brehmer and Dettweiler, and the results which followed the translation of these ideas into practice, had scarcely time to make any major impact on medical thinking when Koch's great announcement came in 1882. It was but natural then that men, surveying the murky waters of current therapy, should now turn to the German genius who had demonstrated the cause in the confident hope that he would place humanity still further in his debt by providing the cure.

Chapter Seven
The Story of Tuberculin

The story of tuberculin is only a brief episode in the history of tuberculosis but it has presented historians with the problem of finding an explanation of the uncharacteristic behaviour of the chief actor in the drama played out in Berlin in 1890–91 with the Western World as audience. Was the uncharacteristic behaviour the result of outside pressures, was it due to a hitherto carefully concealed intellectual arrogance or was it simply an expression of the desire for power?

After his triumph of 1882 Robert Koch was involved for a time in the investigation of cholera in Egypt and India, but in 1884 he published a second and much more exhaustive paper on *The Aetiology of Tuberculosis*. In this he dealt with tuberculosis in many organs and in different animals and took the opportunity to give credit to the work of others which he had borrowed in making his original discovery of the tubercle bacillus.[1] Thereafter he retired behind a barrier of silence which he did not break until 1890 when he addressed the Tenth International Congress of Medicine, assembled in Berlin, on 'Bacteriological Research'. In the course of this address he mentioned that in his study of the tubercle bacillus he had succeeded in producing a substance which held out high hopes for the future.

> My experiments with these substances are likewise not yet completed although I have been occupied with them for nearly a year and I can therefore communicate only this much about them that guinea pigs which, as is well known, are extraordinarily susceptible to tuberculosis, when one subjects them to the operation of such a substance no longer react to inoculation with tuberculosis virus and that in guinea pigs which are already ill with a high grade of general tuberculosis the disease process can be brought to a complete standstill without the body being otherwise

1 Webb, G. B. (1932) Robert Koch. *Ann. med. Hist.* N.S. *4*, 509.

unfavourably influenced by the substance. From these experiments I wish for the present to draw no further conclusions than that the possibility, doubted up to the present time, of making pathogenic bacteria harmless in the living body without injury to the latter, has thereby been proven.[2]

Such a preliminary announcement, guarded though it was, was quite out of keeping with Koch's usual habit. Hitherto he had never spoken until his work was complete and the proof of his thesis established beyond all doubt. Why then did he depart from his customary practice on this occasion especially when dealing with the treatment of tuberculosis, a subject which he must have known full well would produce a strong emotional reaction?

Koch himself never disclosed the reason but an editorial in *The Lancet* later in the year provided a clue:

> Koch, like all scientific men, has his own methods of working, and his own system of declaring his results. He has never yet rushed into print with a discovery until he has been sure of his facts, and all who are in any way acquainted with the circumstances under which Koch was practically compelled by his Government superiors and by his colleagues to make his premature statement at the International Medical Congress in Berlin will sympathise most deeply with him that he was compelled to break through his normal reticence.[3]

This serves as a reminder that Koch was a Government employee and had not, therefore, complete freedom of action.

Any forebodings which he may have had about the effects of this precipitate disclosure were more than fulfilled. So great was the subsequent speculation and so rife was the rumour that on 13 November of that year he felt impelled to publish a fuller account of his discovery under the title *A Further Communication on a Remedy for Tuberculosis*.[4] He opened by saying

> It was originally my intention to complete the research and especially to gain sufficient experience regarding the application of the remedy in practice and its production on a large scale before publishing anything on the subject. But in spite of all precautions, too many accounts have

---

2   Flick, L. F. (1925) *Development of our Knowledge of Tuberculosis*. p. 711. Philadelphia: published by author.
3   Editorial (22 November 1890) *Lancet*, p. 1118.
4   Dr Koch's Own Account of his Remedy. (1890) *Review of Reviews* p. 557.

reached the public, and that in an exaggerated and distorted form, so that it seems imperative, in order to prevent all false impressions, to give at once a review of the subject at the present stage of the inquiry. It is true that this review can, under these circumstances, be only brief and must leave open many important questions.

He then went on to declare that he was unable to make any statement regarding the origin and preparation of the remedy as his researches had not been concluded but he did describe it in the following terms:

The remedy is a brownish transparent liquid, which does not require special care to prevent decomposition. For use this fluid must be more or less diluted, and the dilutions are liable to decomposition if prepared with distilled water: bacterial growths soon develop in them, they become turbid, and are then unfit for use. To prevent this the diluted fluid must be sterilized by heat and preserved under a cotton wool stopper, or more conveniently prepared with a half per cent. solution of phenol.

He added that the remedy was ineffective if given orally and administration had to be by subcutaneous injection. Turning to the question of its mode of action he admitted that as yet this was uncertain since the necessary histological examinations were incomplete but he summarized the existing situation thus:

The remedy does not kill the tubercle bacilli but the tuberculous tissue; and this gives us clearly and definitely the limit that bounds the action of the remedy. It can only influence living tuberculous tissue; it has no effect on dead tissue, as, for example, necrotic cheesy masses, necrotic bones etc., nor has it any effect on tissue made necrotic by the remedy itself. In such masses of dead tissue living tubercle bacilli may possibly still be present, and are either thrown off with the necrosed tissue, or may possibly enter the neighbouring still living tissue under certain circumstances. If the therapeutic activity of the remedy is to be rendered as fruitful as possible, this peculiarity in its mode of action must be carefully observed. In the first instance the living tuberculous tissue must be caused to undergo necrosis, and then everything must be done to remove the dead tissue as soon as possible, as, for instance, by surgical interference. Where this is not possible, and the organism can only help itself in throwing off the tissue slowly, the endangered living tissue must be protected from fresh incursions of the parasites by continuous application of the remedy.

After discussing appropriate dosage schemes Koch proceeded to deal with some of the results of treatment, starting with cases of lupus vulgaris in two of which he claimed that the lupus spots had been brought to complete cicatrization by three or four injections while the remaining cases had improved in proportion to the duration of the treatment. Glandular, bone, and joint tuberculosis had been treated similarly with results which were considered to be equivalent to those of lupus 'a speedy cure in recent and slight cases, slow improvement in severe cases'.

The situation was found to be different in phthisis, where the patients appeared to be much more sensitive to the remedy than those with non-pulmonary disease and consequently the dosage had to be lower. In general, following the initial injection there was some increase in cough and sputum but thereafter the cough grew less while the sputum lost its purulent character and became mucoid. At the same time there was a corresponding improvement in the patient's appearance and general condition.

> Within four to six weeks patients under treatment for the first stage of phthisis were all free from every symptom of disease and might be pronounced cured. Patients with cavities, not yet too highly developed, improved considerably and were almost cured; only in those whose lungs contained many large cavities could no improvement be proved objectively, though even in these cases the expectoration decreased, and the subjective condition improved. These experiences lead me to suppose that phthisis in the beginning can be cured with certainty by this remedy. This sentence requires limitation in so far as at present no conclusive experiences can possibly be brought forward to prove the cure is lasting. Relapses naturally may occur; but it can be assumed that they may be cured as easily and quickly as the first attack.

He then dealt with the reaction to the remedy:

> The healthy human being reacts either not at all or scarcely at all—as we have seen when 0.01 cubic centimetre is used . . . But the case is very different when the disease is tuberculosis; the same dose of 0.01 cubic centimetre injected subcutaneously into the tuberculous patient caused a severe general reaction as well as a local one . . . The general consists in an attack of fever, which, generally beginning with rigors, raises the temperature above 39 degs., often up to 40 degs., and even 41 degs. C.; this is accompanied by pains in the limbs, coughing, great fatigue, often sickness and vomiting. . . The attack usually begins four or five hours after the injection, and lasts for 12 to 15 hours.

Emphasizing that this reaction occurred without exception in all cases where a tuberculous process was present in the organism, after a dose of 0.01 cm³, he continued 'I think I am justified in saying that the remedy will therefore, in future, form an indispensable aid to diagnosis.'

For the moment, however, the world was not interested in the diagnostic uses of tuberculin. The voice of the Master had proclaimed his discovery of the remedy and at the news all Europe erupted. *The Lancet* of November 23rd 1890 in its editorial column gave the subject pride of place.

> The publication by Professor Koch of the method of treating tubercular disease which, as the result of years of patient research, he has discovered, may be taken as evidence that he himself is satisfied of its efficacy.

The writer then went on to note how the announcement was welcome as 'glad tidings of great joy' and to comment on the comparative absence of scepticism among members of a profession who had good reason for being sceptical of alleged specific cures. Koch was also urged to lose no time in making known the details of the preparation of his remedy and so dispose of some of the current rumours amongst which was the suggestion that the German Government was proposing to retain the monopoly of the remedy and thus become 'the proprietary of a vast patent medicine factory.'

Koch's refusal to disclose the nature and method of preparation of his remedy was quite uncharacteristic as indeed was the explanation which he himself provided in an interview which was subsequently published.

> There is very little use my saying just now what the inoculating fluid is or how I have obtained it. It has cost me years of my life and I propose to retain the secret a few weeks longer from publicity . . . Were I to publish now, in the first stage of the discovery, the exact ingredients and method of preparation of the fluid, thousands of medical men, from Moscow to Buenos Ayres, would tomorrow be engaged in concocting it, and injecting it for that matter. Is it far-fetched, then, for me to suppose, as I do, that more than half of these gentleman are incompetent to prepare the fluid which with special study and with special opportunities has taken me years to prepare? Then these experiments might cause incalculable harm to thousands of innocent patients, and at the same time bring into discredit a system of treatment which, I believe, will prove a boon to mankind.[5]

5   *Ibid.* p. 549.

This explanation, if it were the truth, is not greatly to Koch's credit for it appears inexcusable that he should have elaborated on the results of his treatment and at the same time have withheld vital information. He must have known that the refusal to disclose the details of his remedy was bound to alienate ethical medical opinion and, in the long term, to delay the acceptance of his product even should it appear capable of producing the benefits which he had claimed for it. A typical reaction was that of the medical committee of the Brompton Hospital which, at a special meeting held on 20 November, passed unanimously a resolution:

> That the medical officers of this hospital, being desirous to promote in every way the objects for which this institution was founded, will be prepared to take steps to investigate the treatment of consumption as announced by Doctor Koch as soon as the nature of the remedy is before the profession.[6]

It appears probable that political pressure was an important cause of his reticence as a press report stated that on 25 November Dr von Gossler, Minister of Worship and Public Instruction, speaking in the Prussian Diet, said:

> Dr Koch intended to disclose everything he knew frankly and openly, but after a conversation with me in the presence of two witnesses, it was found that he could say nothing upon which others might efficiently produce the remedy. He could say of what the lymph was composed, and describe the method, but it was not possible to demonstrate it. The method is such a difficult and responsible one that it cannot be thought out. It must be arrived at by experiments.

The Minister went on to say that he had requested Dr Koch to disclose the composition of his remedy only partially, so as to render imitation impossible, but that Koch had declared that he could not let the remedy pass out of his hands without having personal control over it. As a result he

> had come to an agreement with Doctor Koch that the remedy should be produced under the management of the State. Even if it was not possible to produce the quantity necessary, yet the whole world would be glad to hear that Prussia had put her stamp upon it. An administrative department would be created which would manage the sale and distribution of the remedy.[7]

6 Editorial. (22 November 1890) *Lancet*, p. 1118.
7 *Review of Reviews* (4) p. 551.

A paragraph in the *Börsen Zeitung*[8] stating that, after making an adequate grant to Dr Koch, the State would undertake the production of his lymph on its own account, provided additional supporting evidence regarding the proposed Government monopoly.

It quickly became clear that, after the initial outburst of excitement and enthusiasm, the profession began to have second thoughts and a further editorial in *The Lancet*[9] exactly one week after it had welcomed the news, spoke of

> an irritational reaction which has taken the form of everything that can be urged, either probable or improbable, against Koch in the first instance and against his remedy in the second.

The writer then proceeded to analyse carefully what Koch had said and what he did not say, concluding that

> Koch holds out hopes of the cure of lupus which he thinks will not recur; of tuberculous glands, of tuberculous joints; and of early phthisis where there is only slight cavity formation; even of laryngeal phthisis; of cases of tubercular meningitis; and of tuberculous disease of others of the serous membranes; but we cannot be astonished that he despairs of being able to effect permanent cures in cases where there are large cavities in the lungs . . . If he is able to make good even a fraction of the promises that he has made, he must be looked upon as one of the greatest benefactors of suffering humanity that the world has seen.

If the medical profession were having second thoughts no such doubts troubled the minds of those tuberculous patients who had heard of the promised land and who, when they could afford it, joined the pilgrimage to Berlin. *The Review of Reviews* devoted the greater part of its issue of December 1890 to the subject and a leading article speaks of the reception of the news of the remedy in the Riviera, at that period still the accepted winter haunt of the tuberculous patient.

> Hence through all that region the news that the German scientist had discovered a cure for consumption must have sounded as the news of the advent of Jesus of Nazareth in a Judaean village. The whole country was moved to meet him. His fame went throughout the whole region round about, and telegrams in the newspapers announced that all the sleeping cars had been engaged for months to convey the consumptives of the Riviera to the inclement latitude of Berlin.

8   *Ibid.* p. 560.
9   Editorial (29 November 1890) *Lancet*, p. 1168.

The same issue included an assessment of the remedy by Arthur Conan Doyle, who had gone to Berlin, which was to prove uncannily accurate.

It must never be lost sight of that Koch has never claimed that his fluid kills the tubercle bacillus. On the contrary it has no effect on it but destroys the low form of tissue in the meshes of which the baccilli lie. Should the tissue slough in the case of lupus, or be expelled in the sputum in the case of phthisis and should it contain in its meshes all the bacilli, then it would be possible to hope for a complete cure. When one considers, however, the number and the minute size of these deadly organisms, and the evidence that the lymphatics as well as the organs are affected by them, it is evident that it will only be in very exceptional cases that the bacilli are all expelled.

Doyle summarised his views thus:

There can be no question that it forms an admirable aid to diagnosis. Tubercle, and tubercle alone responds to its action, so that in all cases where the exact nature of a complaint is doubtful, a single injection is enough to determine whether it is scrofulous, lupus, phthisical, or in any way tuberculous. This alone is a very important addition to the art of medicine. Of its curative action in lupus there can be no question, though I have heard Doctor Koeler, the Berlin specialist upon skin affections, express a doubt as to the permanancy of the cicatrix . . . In the case of true phthisis of the lungs, which is of more immediate importance in these islands, the evidence is so slight that we can only regard it as an indication and a hope, rather than a proof. It is obvious that the difficulty of getting rid of the tubercular matter is enormously increased when the diseased products are buried deeply in a vital organ. It may prove that even here the specific action of the remedy may triumph over the degenerative process, but it would be an encouraging of false hopes to pretend that this result was in any way assured.[10]

A note of warning was being sounded now in the chief clinical centres. In Vienna, Billroth hoped that the remedy, when carefully used, might arrest the progress of consumption but did not believe that it could ever cure it while he could envisage circumstances in which its use might do immeasurable harm. Kowalski, Chief of the Bacteriological Institute for Army Physicians in Vienna was most guarded when disease of the lungs' was in question. Schmitz from Antwerp reported that, though it was said that the remedy slowly

10   *Review of Reviews* (4) p. 556.

cured lupus, till now not a single case had been cured completely while as regards pulmonary phthisis the remedy was still doubtful.[11]

It was clear that the consensus opinion of those who were reporting results with the remedy failed to support a number of Koch's claims for its therapeutic action although there was fairly general endorsement of its value in diagnosis. A further and telling blow was struck when Virchow entered the lists to report his pathological findings in cases where tuberculin had been used. Sixteen of these had had pulmonary tuberculosis; one had had non-pulmonary disease. Virchow found

> evidence of irritation in the tissues everywhere and of new inflammatory change in many places. In old lung cavities the granular layers of the superficial border were very red and frequently there was haemorrhagic infiltration of the cavity wall. In the deeper layers there were positive inflammatory processes with active proliferation on a large scale. There was also swelling of the bronchial and mediastinal glands such as occurs when there is acute irritation. Most of the cases of ulcerative phthisis had extensive recent changes in the lungs and pleura while there were some miliary tubercles noted in the serous membranes which appeared to be of recent origin and to have developed subsequent to the injections.[12]

In 1891 it became clear even to Koch that he must disclose the nature of the remedy and its mode of preparation. The disclosure was made in a paper in which he reported further favourable results, declared that the poor results of others must have been due to their selection of far-advanced cases for study and declined to entertain the suggestion that the remedy directly furthered the tuberculous process. He went on to describe the 'Koch phenomenon' showing that a tuberculous animal offered much resistance to a new infection although often unable to overcome the original disease, and concluded that something must act upon the tuberculous process 'in a curative manner', this something being a 'soluble substance which was dissolved out of the bodies of the bacilli by the fluids surrounding them.' This brought him to the climax of his work, namely, the separation of this curative substance from the bacilli, and to his announcement that 'the remedy with which the new method of treating tuberculosis is carried out is, therefore, a glycerine extract of a pure culture of tubercle bacilli'.[13]

11   *Ibid.* p. 560.
12   Flick, L. F. (2) pp. 724–5.
13   *Ibid.* pp. 719–21.

But the disclosure had come too late and had not been couched in terms which might have mollified the critics. An editorial in the *British Medical Journal* was bitterly hostile.

> It was hoped that at last, by a full judicial account of the methods of preparation of tuberculin ... Dr. Koch would make a welcome and satisfactory, if tardy, requital for the patient long-suffering of his fellow medical men and his bacteriological *confrères*. We are sorry to confess that it is not in our power to declare that this requital has been made ... It is impossible for us not to feel that the tone of the remarks with which he prefaces this description is most unhappy. Much of the opposition which the use of tuberculin has encountered at the hands of the profession at large is due to the exceptional methods which Doctor Koch was ill-advised enough to adopt in the first instance in publishing his discovery to the world. Throughout this critical period of his history, bacteriologists ... have as a body supported him patiently and loyally. And now they are reproached for their inability to follow out his method upon their own initiative ... We think it probable that the results of these ungracious remarks will be to alienate from Professor Koch much of the sympathy and the support which he has hitherto received from his fellow-workers. As to the method itself, it is one well known to bacteriologists, involving no special difficulties. We are bound to confess on reading it that there appears to us to be little necessity for having kept it a secret so long. The method of cultivation of the tubercle bacilli which Professor Koch adopts is one we owe to the labours of the French bacteriologists.[14]

The wild, uncritical enthusiasm which had greeted the introduction of tuberculin into therapy had now given way to a steady, progressive disillusionment. It soon became obvious that it killed more patients than it helped and in a relatively short period of time it was discredited practically everywhere. Koch himself maintained his belief in it and produced several variations of tuberculin which he hoped might improve its therapeutic potential but he was unable to satisfy his critics. In a few years it had been discarded by all apart from a very few isolated enthusiasts who continued to use it in much reduced dosage. At this level it proved harmless but it was notable that these enthusiasts failed to convince their professional colleagues of the realities of its alleged benefits. So tuberculin treatment passed into history to become a perpetual reminder to future generations of the perils of premature publicity and of exaggerated claims of clinical success.

14   Editorial (31 October 1891) *Br. med. J.* pp. 954–5.

Nevertheless, Koch's work on tuberculin had not been in vain since through it he had provided medicine with one of its most useful diagnostic aids in the form of a testing substance which is still employed throughout the world. He himself moved on to explore other fields, becoming in 1891 Director of the newly created Institute of Infectious Diseases in Berlin from which he was to make valuable contributions to the control of cholera, typhoid and sleeping sickness and to be rewarded with a Nobel Prize in 1905.

Chapter Eight
The Early Sanatoria

The history of tuberculosis after 1882 shows how increasing effort was being devoted to treatment, effort which was intensified after it became clear that tuberculin had no place in therapeutics. The effect found practical expression in a two-pronged attack, the indirect approach inherent in sanatorium treatment with its emphasis on fresh air and general bodily rest and the direct approach in which rest was applied locally to the diseased lung by a series of surgical manoeuvres of varying ingenuity and severity. Both methods had been conceived and tentatively initiated before Koch's discovery but this, acting as a stimulus, brought them sharply into the foreground where they were pursued with increasing vigour during the years which intervened before the outbreak of war in 1914 diverted the world's thoughts and energies to other fields.

In Germany the work begun by Brehmer and Dettweiler was carried on by Otto Walther who established a sanatorium at Nordrach in the Black Forest at an altitude of 1500 feet. Walther believed in keeping his patients in bed until they were afebrile and had regained some of their lost weight. Thereafter they were started on graduated exercise, which consisted of walking only and which was prescribed with great precision. He considered an adequate diet to be of prime importance and to him this meant a minimum of three very full meals each day which had to be consumed regardless of appetite while he was the first to introduce the preprandial rest hour, thus setting a pattern which was to be followed in British (though not in Continental) sanatoria for very many years. He was convinced of the need for strict discipline and insisted on rigid adherence to the sanatorium rules; quite minor infringements of these could result in dismissal.

Walther and Nordrach, although the former was viewed with reserve by his German confrères who considered his methods unorthodox and failed to understand why he published so little, rapidly acquired an international reputation. At one stage in 1904, 14 different nationalities were represented among his patients of whom over 50 per cent were British.[1] But possibly the greatest tribute to the man and his work was provided by many of the sanatoria which opened in Britain around the beginning of the century and which adopted not only his methods but also in some instances the name of his sanatorium, styling themselves Nordrach-in-Wales or Nordrach-on-Mendip according to location.

In the United States the therapy of tuberculosis was virtually non-existent until the advent of Edward Livingstone Trudeau who had this deficiency brought forcibly to his notice while engaged in his own personal battle with the disease. The descendant of a French family which had settled and prospered in Louisiana, he had had a somewhat restless youth followed by an undistinguished student career at Columbia University where he graduated in medicine in March 1871.[2] Later that year he entered into practice with a prominent New York physician, an arrangement which virtually guaranteed him a secure and lucrative future, but these dreams of success were rudely shattered in February 1873 when, after a series of attacks of fever without obvious cause, he consulted a senior colleague and was told that he had active tuberculosis involving the upper two-thirds of his left lung. Such a diagnosis at that period was tantamount to a death sentence and this was clearly in Trudeau's mind when he decided to go to the Adirondack mountains in the north of New York State—not that he thought that the climate would be in any way beneficial but because the wildness of the area and its forests appealed to him and, as he put it, 'It seemed to meet a longing I had for rest and the peace of the great wilderness.'

His objective was Saranac Lake, where he spent most of his time out doors but wisely kept his exertions to the minimum. Over the succeeding months his health steadily improved but deteriorated again on his return to New York in the autumn and by May 1874 he was back at Saranac as ill as before. He now came to the conclusion that the Adirondacks represented his only hope of survival; in November 1876 his family joined him at Saranac and the first step towards a great project had been taken. With returning health and strength came the wish that the benefits which he had derived from life in the Adirondacks could be extended to others, particularly the poorer members

1 Pearson, S. V. (1946) *Men, Medicine and Myself.* p. 32. London: Museum Press.
2 Meade, G. M. (1972) Edward Livingstone Trudeau, M. D. *Tubercle 53*, 299.

of the community whose need was greatest. The chief obstacle in the path of realization of this wish was the lack of suitable and cheap accommodation, an obstacle which remained insuperable until 1882 when, after reading an account of a visit to Gorbersdorf in an English journal, Trudeau decided that the needs of his prospective patients could be met by the construction of a few simple cottages at Saranac Lake. He solicited subscriptions from all his friends and from anyone else whom he thought would help, displaying a latent talent as a mendicant that was to stand him in good stead in the future. Not only were patients never charged the full cost of their treatment at Saranac but in addition a substantial endowment fund was created.[2]

During the winter of 1884–85 the first cottage was completed and in February 1885 the first two patients were admitted. From such a beginning grew the Trudeau sanatorium and later there was to stand beside it the Saranac laboratory. Under Trudeau's direction and guidance these two establishments achieved international fame, converting Saranac Lake into a focal point, whence knowledge of tuberculosis was disseminated all over the world. The extent of his influence on the antituberculosis campaign in the United States may be gauged from the fact that by 1925 there were 261 physicians who had either cured or studied at Saranac and thereafter gone into sanatorium work. These men were scattered throughout America in every state of the Union except six and in every province in Canada.[3]

A further notable contributor to the growth of the sanatorium movement in the United States was Vincent Y. Bowditch of Boston whose vision was responsible for the creation of the first state sanatorium for tuberculosis, which opened at Rutland, Massachusetts, in 1899, and for the establishment of the Sharon sanatorium for working women in 1891.[4] The establishment of these two institutions was to have a profound influence on the later development of public health programmes for the care of the tuberculous by demonstrating that a state government could and would assume responsibility for the building of sanatoria if public opinion could be aroused sufficiently to secure legislation. In addition the results obtained at Sharon sanatorium showed that tuberculosis could be treated successfully, even at sea level and in a supposedly unfavourable climate, thus providing

3 Lyman, D. R. (1925) The influence of Trudeau on the sanatorium movement. *J. Outdoor Life* 22, 28.
4 Jacobs, P. H. (1932) The control of tuberculosis in the United States. *N.Y. Nat. Tuberc. Ass.* p. 18.

an answer to those sceptics in other states who were only too ready to discourage the expenditure of public funds for sanatorium treatment on the grounds that sites providing suitable climatic conditions were not available within the borders of the state.

In Britain the first institution reserved exclusively for the open air treatment of pulmonary tuberculosis was the Royal Victoria Hospital founded in Edinburgh in 1894. The movement soon spread beyond Edinburgh and in 1896 the National Hospital for Consumption was opened at Newcastle, County Wicklow, while in the west of Scotland William Quarrier, a noted Glasgow philanthropist, was the moving spirit behind the opening of the Consumption Sanatoria of Scotland at Bridge of Weir, Renfrewshire, in 1897. Nordrach-on-Dee sanatorium at Banchory, Kincardineshire was opened in 1900, Mundesley sanatorium in Norfolk quickly followed, while 1904 saw the opening of the Brompton Hospital sanatorium at Frimley, Surrey, and of the King Edward VII sanatorium, Midhurst, Sussex, both destined to become famous centres of treatment in the years ahead.

In Switzerland the mountain resort of Davos was developing a 'sanatorium industry' with the aid of skilful publicity extolling the alleged special benefits of altitude and fresh mountain air and in France sanatoria under the direction of Küss at Agincourt and of Dumarest at Hauteville had been established in 1900, the year which also saw the opening of Mesnalien sanatorium in Norway and of Vejlefjord in Denmark.

During the opening years of the twentieth century, the sanatorium movement can be said to have got well off the ground and by 1912–13 there were in Britain 52 sanatoria or kindred institutions dedicated to the open air treatment of pulmonary tuberculosis.[5] By and large these adhered to the regimen favoured by Walther in which the patient was kept in bed until he was afebrile, when it was permissible to begin walking exercise—provided that this was meticulously prescribed and controlled.

There was one notable deviant from this general acceptance of Walther's programme in the person of Marcus Paterson who, early in 1905, had been appointed medical superintendent of the newly opened Brompton Hospital sanatorium at Frimley. Here he made some pertinent observations, one of which was that a proportion of

5 Kelynack, T. N. (ed.) *The Tuberculosis Year Book and Sanatoria Annual* (1913–14) pp. xxi–xxii. London: John Bale, Sons & Danielsson.

the patients who had been employed in heavy manual labour up to the time of their admission had, despite this, remained in remarkably good general condition. From this he argued that if such patients

> under adverse circumstances, and without any medical guidance, could act thus without apparent injury they might, under ideal conditions and with the work carefully graduated in accordance with their physical state, to be able to undertake useful labour.[6]

In his proposal to replace the gentle walk of Walther by more strenuous endeavours Paterson believed that

> manual work should be of great advantage to patients undergoing treatment in a sanatorium, as, first, it would do much to meet the objections that members of the working class are liable to have their energy sapped and to acquire lazy habits by such treatment; secondly, it would make them more resistant to the disease, by improving their physical condition; and thirdly, would enable them by its effect upon their muscles to return to their work immediately after their discharge.

He devised grades of work the lightest of which consisted in carrying baskets of mould for the sanatorium lawns while the top grade entailed the use of a pickaxe for six hours daily. Throughout, of course, he observed his patients carefully and anyone showing a rise of temperature was immediately returned to bed rest. Paterson believed that his patients benefited considerably from this graduated labour programme and evolved a theory to explain the benefit in which he postulated the inoculation of the patient with his own tuberculin as the result of the physical work. He looked upon a rise of temperature occurring while a patient was working as evidence of such an 'auto-inoculation' and convinced himself that thereafter that patient made better progress.

Whatever dubious advantages may have accrued to the patient from these labours there is no doubt that the sanatorium was a major beneficiary. Powell and Hartley record with pride that

> the patients have carried out much useful work at the sanatorium, although many of them had before been engaged in clerical and sedentary occupations . . . A reservoir capable of holding 500 000 gallons has been excavated and concreted. Trees have been cut down and sawn into firewood, the sanatorium has been painted, a kitchen garden trenched and cultivated, and the grounds kept in order.[7]

6   Paterson, M. S. (1908) Graduated labour in pulmonary tuberculosis. *Lancet 1*, 216.
7   Powell, D. & Hartley, P. H.-S. (1921) *Diseases of the Lungs and Pleurae*. p. 611. London: H. K. Lewis.

The vigour with which Paterson propounded his thesis allied to his considerable personal charm found him many adherents who overlooked, as he did, the fact that his proposals involved keeping 'toxic' patients on exercise. Many also failed to appreciate that his patients constituted a selected group who had been carefully sifted by the consulting staff at Brompton Hospital before being recommended for admission to Frimley, while he himself seems to have remained unaware that the temperature readings upon which his scheme depended were not wholly reliable being often subject to adjustment by the patient in his desire to be allowed up again.[8]

While British therapeutics were being influenced by Paterson and his 'autoinoculation' theory opinion elsewhere was moving steadily in the direction of more rest, even when afebrile, as advocated by Pratt[9] in the United States where he had the authoritative support of Trudeau and Lawrason Brown. It was not until 1923, when Clive Rivière, assessing the results of rest therapy as practised by Pratt in America and autoinoculation therapy as introduced by Paterson in Britain, convincingly demonstrated the superiority of the former, that British sanatoria were freed from the shackles of graduated labour to turn to the therapeutic regimen of rest which was so steadily gaining ground.

Initially these British sanatoria were either private ventures run for profit or voluntary institutions supported by charitable donations, and, admirable though their work may have been, they were able to accommodate only a fraction of those in need of their services. Within a few years from the beginning of the century it was becoming clear that the battle against the disease constituted a national problem, the solution of which was beyond the resources of private enterprise and voluntary effort. With this realization came the call for government action but before considering the inauguration of the resulting legislative programme it is necessary to step back again into the nineteenth century to trace the tentative beginnings of chest radiology and also the origins of the collapse therapy of pulmonary tuberculosis, two developments destined to go hand in hand in the years which lay ahead and to usher in a phase of active treatment to supplement the passive regime of rest and exercise on which sanatorium life was based.

8 Pearson, S. V. (1) p. 81.
9 Pratt, J. H. (1932) The development of the rest treatment of pulmonary tuberculosis. *New Engl. J. Med. 206*, 64.

Chapter Nine
The Advent of Radiology

Although the discovery of X-rays by Wilhelm Conrad Röntgen in 1895 was accorded a mixed reception there was not the outright and universal chorus of disparagement and condemnation which had greeted most previous discoveries of similar import. It is true that at Röntgen's memorable lecture before the Würzburg Physical Medical Society on the night of 23 January 1896, Professor Schonbrun had intervened to warn the audience against too much optimism 'since the method scarcely promised to be of much, if any, value in the diagnosis of internal disturbances';[1] while one month later an editorial in the *Boston Medical and Surgical Journal* commented 'that the discovery, whatever future it may have before it, will fall short of our over-sanguine hopes is almost inevitable'. But in spite of the forebodings of the professional sceptics and pessimists world-wide interest had been aroused by the discovery of this ray with its possible use in diagnosis and perhaps even in treatment, so that the more imaginative physicians and scientists proposed to explore the matter for themselves and without delay.

In Britain, on 18 March 1897, at a meeting held at 20, King William Street, Strand, W.C., the premises of the Medical Defence Union, a group of interested physicians and surgeons formed The X-ray Society, destined to become the first radiological society in the world. At a subsequent meeting the basis of membership was extended to include non-medical scientists and the name of the Society amended to The Röntgen Society. Silvanus Thompson, F.R.S., Professor of Physics in the City and Guilds of London Technical College, became the Society's first President, delivering his Presidential address on 5 November 1897, when he opened with the dramatic sentence: 'November the eighth, 1895, will ever be memorable in the history of

1 Brown, L. (1941) *The Story of Clinical Pulmonary Tuberculosis.* pp. 214–15. Baltimore: Williams & Wilkins.

science. On that day a light which, so far as human observation goes, never was on land or sea, was first observed'.[2]

The possible use of the new discovery in the diagnosis and management of pulmonary tuberculosis appeared to arouse the interest of the general public even at this early stage, as an annotation in the *Lancet* of 15 February 1896, indicated:

> All sorts of crude ideas seem to be current as to the application in medicine of the new radiations or X-rays. We had an enquiry from a lay correspondent last week as to where the apparatus producing these new radiations could be obtained as it was wanted for a case of consumption.[3]

The public's reaction also had its lighter moments: a few weeks after the announcement of the discovery one London firm was alleged to have advertised the sale of X-ray-proof underclothing; while, in February 1896, it is reported that a Bill to prohibit the use of X-rays in opera glasses in theatres was introduced in the Legislative Assembly of the State of New Jersey.[4]

In the United States the pioneer in the employment of radiology in the diagnosis and management of pulmonary tuberculosis was Francis H. Williams of Boston. Throughout 1896 he had conducted X-ray examinations on 400 patients, the majority of whom were suffering from some form of respiratory disease including more than 100 cases of pulmonary tuberculosis, and in the latter he had

> found a correspondence between the physical signs and the X-ray examinations in a considerable number of cases; in certain cases this instrument showed that the disease was more extensive than the physical examination indicated; *in others it showed an increase in density in the lungs earlier than was detected by the physical examination; and while in some of these no signs in the lungs were detected prior to those found by the fluoroscope, in others, although one lung was ascertained by the physical examination to be seriously involved, its companion was not suspected until the x-ray examination revealed its increased density.*[5]

These pioneering endeavours and opinions naturally encountered

2   Thompson, S. (1897) *Archs Roentg. Ray.* 2, 23.
3   The New Photography (1896) *Lancet 1*, 432.
4   Brown, L. (1) p. 214.
5   Williams, F. H. (1897) The Röntgen ray in thoracic disease. *Am. J. med. Sci. 114*, 665.

resistance and, in a discussion of a paper by Williams, F. S. Shattuck is credited with the remark:

> Frank Williams has just shown you some plates and tells you that the heart is here and the lung is here. Now I can't see a thing in these plates, and to be truthful I don't think that he can.[6]

During these early stages opinion was divided on the relative merits of fluoroscopy and radiography. The former was less time-consuming, less expensive and (a boon to the inexperienced) did not show up the normal lung markings which so confused those unfamiliar with radiographic interpretation. Minor of Ashville, Tennessee, a vehement supporter of fluoroscopy, claimed that the radiograph furnished such a wealth of detail that interpretation became too difficult, a view which Cole demolished by remarking that it would be just as rational to discard the high power microscope because of the increased detail which it provided.

The argument was eventually resolved conclusively in favour of radiography as technical improvements permitted shorter exposures and better quality films, but even before then X-ray examination had been revealing tuberculous lesions, unsuspected on physical examination, with sufficient frequency to stimulate constructive thought and F. H. Williams soon made powerful converts in the persons of Edward L. Trudeau and H. P. Loomis, the Trudeau Sanatorium becoming one of the first in the United States to use X-ray examination for all patients. Improvements in technique continued and by 1910 Lewis G. Cole, who had been appointed consulting radiologist to the New York Board of Health, was asserting that not only had radiology solved the problem of the diagnosis of incipient tuberculosis but it had also made it possible to determine with a reasonable degree of certainty the variety of the lesion, whether it represented active or inactive disease and, with absolute certainty, whether the process was advancing, static or resolving.[7]

In France valuable exploratory work was carried out by L. Bouchard[8] and A. Béclère. The latter, in 1901, was declaring that 'examination by radioscope and radiography supersedes all other methods'[9]

6 Brown, L. (1) p. 216.
7 Cole, L. G. (1910) The radiographic diagnosis and classification of early pulmonary tuberculosis. *Am. J. med. Sci. 140*, 29.
8 Bouchard, L. (1896) Application de la radioscopie au diagnostic des maladies du thorax. *Rev. Tuberc. 4*, 273.
9 Béclere, A. (1902) On the technique of the application of the Röntgen rays in the diagnosis of tuberculosis. *Trans. Br. Congr. Tuberc.* 1901, *3*, 278.

although five years later, in 1906, his distinguished compatriot, Edouard Rist, is recorded as still adhering to the belief that careful physical examination was the most effective means of diagnosing early tuberculosis.[10]

In Britain, although Röntgen's work attracted much interest, as illustrated by the prompt formation of the Röntgen Society, no-one appeared to be in any immediate hurry to investigate its diagnostic possibilities in thoracic disease apart from John Macintyre, the Glasgow laryngologist, who employed X-rays to localize a small coin wedged in a patient's oesophagus.[11] In 1901, when the British Congress on Tuberculosis met in London, a short 'Discussion on the use of the Röntgen rays in the diagnosis of pulmonary tuberculosis' was fitted into the programme. The opening speaker, Hugh Walsham, cast some doubt on the ability of radiology to reveal the really early tuberculous lesion but Béclere, the French pioneer, who followed him, spoke with enthusiasm of its potentialities in this field which, he claimed, were now universally recognized. This, unfortunately, was still far from being the case and years were to elapse before such wide recognition was accorded in Britain.

One man who foresaw almost immediately the contribution which radiology could make to the study of respiratory disease was a young and still relatively unknown Scottish physician who, without further ado, set about exploiting these possibilities to the full. David Lawson had noted the almost total lack of sanatoria in Britain, particularly for private patients, who consequently betook themselves to Germany and Switzerland. He visited Walther at Nordrach, studied his sanatorium and its methods, and concluded that there was nothing in either which he could not satisfactorily reproduce. He selected for his project a site on the southern slope of a hill overlooking the village of Banchory in the valley of the Aberdeenshire Dee, built his sanatorium and opened it in 1900 under the name of Nordrach-on-Dee, a choice of title which produced a vigorous but unavailing protest from Walther.[12]

Lawson had the foresight and wisdom to include a Röntgen ray apparatus in his basic equipment and to appoint an electrotherapeutist, Hill Crombie, to his staff: both were employed to good purpose. Lawson's first communication on radiology in chest disease was

10 Brown, L. (1) p. 222.
11 Macintyre, J. (1896) Röntgen rays in laryngeal surgery. *J. Lar. 10*, 231.
12 Lawson, D. Personal Communication.

presented before the Edinburgh Medico-Chirurgical Society on 3 June 1903 and was published in the *Lancet* on 25 July that year.[13] Illustrating his paper with reproductions of X-ray plates he discussed appearances such as the 'roof-tiling' of the ribs in association with unresolved pneumonia and lobar collapse, cardiac enlargement with emphysema, pleural effusion and pleural thickening and, in tuberculosis, chronic fibroid phthisis and cavitation. Finally, for good measure, he added a case of thoracic actinomycosis. In 1902 Gardiner,[14] writing in the *Scottish Medical Journal*, had complained that 'the use of X-rays in the diagnosis of pulmonary tuberculosis has now spread to many lands but as yet comparatively little has been done in Scotland'. Lawson's work was the answer to this plaint, and indeed, for a time it seemed as though he had the field almost to himself.

His second paper appeared in *The Practitioner* in 1906[15] and his third in that same journal in 1913.[16] In this last he voiced his dissatisfaction with the laggard acceptance of radiology as a major diagnostic advance in diseases of the chest, castigating in particular the far from inconsiderable body of physicians who still failed to utilize X-rays in the diagnosis of obscure lung lesions. He reserved for special condemnation the physician who, without a preceding X-ray, thrust a trocar into the chest as his sole means of differentiating between lobar consolidation and pleural effusion. In the field of diagnostic radiology Lawson was undoubtedly well ahead of his contemporaries and the speciality of chest medicine suffered a very real loss when in 1916 he elected to retire from clinical practice in order to develop his other role, that of a director in his family's business.

It would seem justifiable to conclude that Lawson's work had given a clear indication of the pathway to be followed in developing and expanding chest radiology but the response to his call was, to say the least of it, sluggish. *The Tuberculosis Year Book* and *Sanatoria Annual* for 1913–14 published the results of a questionnaire designed to provide information about the facilities available for the tuberculous patient in Britain.[17] Seventeen local authorities reported that they were

13 Lawson, D. & Hill Crombie, R. (1903) Röntgen rays in the diagnosis of lung disease. *Lancet*, 25 July.
14 Gardiner, F. (1902) X-rays as a diagnosis agent in phthisis pulmonalis. *Scott. med. J. 11*, 402.
15 Lawson, D. (1906) X-rays in the diagnosis of lung disease. *Practitioner* (extra number on X-rays) 17.
16 Lawson, D. (1913) X-rays in the diagnosis of lung disease. *Practitioner 90*, 53.
17 Kelynack, T. N. (1913–14) *The Tuberculosis Year Book and Sanatoria Annual*. London: John Bale, Sons & Danielsson.

operating tuberculosis dispensaries, of which only five had X-ray equipment, while of the 96 sanatoria investigated only seven had provided an X-ray department. No authoritative lead appeared to be coming from the seats of learning and Sir Robert Philip, shortly to become professor of tuberculosis at Edinburgh, delivered an address to the Glasgow Southern Medical Society on 20 March 1913 during which he dealt with problems of diagnosis without making any reference to radiology.[18] For him all diagnostic requirements were met by clinical examination and tuberculin testing. Even by 1920, a quarter of a century after Röntgen's discovery, there were still deficiencies; Vere Pearson, senior physician at Mundesley sanatorium and one of the pioneers of artificial pneumothorax treatment in Britain, recalls in his reminiscences a visit which he paid that year to North Wales to seek advice from Morriston Davies before installing an X-ray apparatus at Mundesley.[19]

It is difficult to escape the conclusion that the recognition of radiology as an integral part of the investigation of any case of respiratory disease was impeded by the deeply entrenched resistance of many senior and influential physicians. Accustomed to having their *ex cathedra* pronouncements on the results of their physical examination accepted as Holy Writ, their opposition to any innovation which might produce evidence incompatible with these findings and thus cast a slur upon their competence was implacable. The measure of this opposition is well illustrated in the sixth edition of the standard text-book of the day *On Diseases of the Lungs and Pleurae* by Sir Douglas Powell and Sir Percival Horton-Smith Hartley published in 1921. These distinguished authors, both physicians to the Brompton Hospital, maintained 'that our experience, then, is that in early cases of phthisis the diagnosis can, as a rule, be made by physical signs before the appearance of characteristic X-ray changes'. They continued:

'The following case in which the X-rays proved helpful in detecting a deep-seated area of tuberculous consolidation before the occurrence of physical signs or the discovery of tubercle bacilli in the sputum appears worth recording, though we must emphasize that the case is an exceptional one . . . Such cases are, however, quite rare and their occasional

18   Philip, R. W. (1937) *Collected papers on Tuberculosis.* p. 147. London: Oxford University Press.
19   Pearson, S. V. (1946) *Men, Medicine and Myself.* p. 98. London: Museum Press.

occurrence does not alter our conclusion that only exceptionally can we expect assistance from the x-rays in the diagnosis of phthisis.'[20]*

X-ray examination as an essential factor in the diagnosis and management of tuberculosis received a powerful boost from the increasing use of artificial pneumothorax and by 1922 L. S. T. Burrell and A. S. Macnalty were writing in a Medical Research Council *Report on Artificial Pneumothorax* that they considered the use of X-rays to be essential not only to provide evidence on the state of the lungs before treatment but also to assess the degree of collapse, the presence and extent of pleural adhesions and the occurrence of any complicating effusion.[21] By 1925 the thoracic surgeons were becoming at home in the therapeutic field and demanding the X-rays even before they saw the patient, a piece of clinical heresy which shook the medical establishment to its foundations, and before the 1930s were reached routine X-ray examination of cases of pulmonary tuberculosis had become a fact of life.

Thus, after a quarter of a century, Lawson's opinions were vindicated: but even he could hardly have been expected to foresee the immense contribution which radiology had yet to make, nor to visualize the advent of mass miniature radiography which was to play such a vital role in programmes directed towards the control of tuberculosis in the middle decades of the century.

---

* Even the technological advances of later years failed to persuade Sir Percival Horton-Smith Hartley to amend his outlook. In 1937, although long retired from active hospital work, he still maintained a clinical interest in a selected number of his former tuberculous patients. One of these, who was due to see him, asked the writer, then First Assistant Medical Officer at the King Edward VII Sanatorium, Midhurst, to X-ray his chest and to allow him to take the film with him to his appointment so that the most recent information might be available at the time of consultation. The film was duly presented to Sir Percival whose *riposte* was a pained letter pointing out that since the distribution of the X-ray changes did not correspond with that of his physical signs it was obvious that the wrong film must have been sent and could the correct one now please be forwarded?

20   Powell, R. D. & Hartley, P. H.-S. (1921) *On Diseases of the Lungs and Pleurae.* pp. 576–8. London: H. K. Lewis.
21   Burrell, L. S. T. & Macnalty, A. S. (1922) *Medical Research Council Report on Artificial Pneumothorax.* London: H.M.S.O.

Chapter Ten
Collapse Therapy

The results obtained by the orthodox treatment of the day were usually poor and always uncertain and were bound to lead more venturesome spirits into the consideration of some form of direct assault on the diseased lung.

The first suggestion of this appears to have come from Georgius Baglivi who, in 1696, wrote in his *De Praxi Medica*, Book ii, Chapter xi:

> A phthisick arising from an ulcer in the lungs is commonly branded as incurable, upon the plea that the ulcer is internal and occult, and cannot be cleansed like other external ulcers. But why do they not make it their business to find out the true situation of the ulcer, and make an incision accordingly between the ribs, to the end that proper remedies may be conveyed to it? For my part, I know no reason why that should lie neglected. About seven years ago when I was at Padua, a man received a wound in the right side of his breast that reached to the lung, and employing an able surgeon had an incision made between the ribs to the length of six fingers breadth, in order to discover the situation of the wound in the lung which was perfectly cured in two months time with vulneraries apply'd with tents and with syringing. Now practitioners ought to use the same piece of diligence in curing a phthisical ulcer in the lungs, lest the scroll of incurable diseases should grow too long to the infinite disgrace of the profession. Believe me, gentlemen, assiduous thought and use improves and whets the mind, but sloth and despair breaks its edge.[1]

There is no evidence that Baglivi did more than exhort his contemporaries to greater effort and although Alexander has noted that sporadic reports appeared in the literature of the eighteenth century either advising incision of the chest or recording favourable results

1 Baglivi, G. (1696) Quoted by Balboni, G. M. (1935). The development of the treatment of pulmonary tuberculosis from 1696 to the present time. *New Engl. J. Med.* 1020.

following wounds in the chest in patients with pulmonary symptoms, it is not clear whether, at that stage, any distinction was made between drainage of the pleural cavity and collapse of the lung.[2]

The first firm reference to the possibility of collapse therapy was made almost casually by M. Bourru, the librarian to the Faculty of Medicine in Paris, who in 1770 undertook the translation into French of Ebenezer Gilchrist's book *The Use of Sea Voyages in Medicine: Particularly in a Consumption with Observations on that Disease*. Gilchrist in his text made no reference to any idea of surgical treatment, but Bourru in his translator's preface suggests

> that if it were only the movement, as one says, which is opposed to the healing and cicatrization of the ulcer . . . one might be able to remedy this by an operation similar to that which one performs in the case of empyema. In this an opening is made into the side of the chest that is diseased. It is known that as soon as air is introduced into one of the cavities of the chest where lie the lungs, the lung on this side collapses and no longer plays a part; the other lung then alone carries on respiration. This communication of the cavity of the chest where lies the diseased lung with the exterior air, lasts until nature, aided by external remedies, has been able to cicatrize the ulcer, assuming always that the trouble is local and not habitual or scattered throughout the body.[3]

This suggestion by Bourru excited no immediate comment and indeed appears to have passed unnoticed until 1820 when it was discovered by J. P. Maygrier who (having erroneously attributed the notion to Gilchrist himself rather than to his translator) lost no time in making his own attitude clear with the opinion that 'the uselessness and danger of such an operation ought to make it forever rejected from the domain of the art'.[4]

The first physician to apply his mind wholeheartedly and earnestly to the possibility of a therapeutic pneumothorax was James Carson. Carson, a Scot, had begun his university career with the intention of entering the church but subsequently turned to medicine, graduating at the University of Edinburgh in 1799. Later he settled in Liverpool where, on the title page of his earliest publication, *An Enquiry into the Causes of the Motion of the Blood* in 1815, he is described as 'Physician to

2 Alexander, J. (1937) *The Collapse Therapy of Pulmonary Tuberculosis*. p. 23. Springfield, Illinois: C. C. Thomas.
3 Brown, L. (1941) *The Story of Clinical Pulmonary Tuberculosis*. pp. 235–6. Baltimore: Williams & Wilkins.
4 *Ibid*. p. 236.

the Workhouse Fever Hospital and the Asylum for Pauper Lunatics at Liverpool, and in charge of the Military Hospital at that Place'. Thereafter he is known to have built up an extensive private practice yet he continued to find time for serious scientific study and was able, from well-conducted and original physiological experiments, to establish clearly and correctly the part played in the mechanics of respiration by the elasticity of the lungs. In his paper *On the Elasticity of the Lungs* after describing his animal experiments, he continued:

> Two powers are therefore concerned in regulating the movements and in varying the dimensions and form of the diaphragm. Of these powers the one is permanent and equable, the other variable and exerted at intervals. The contractile power of the diaphragm, when fully exerted, is evidently much stronger than its antagonist, the resilience of the lungs; but the latter not being subject to exhaustion, takes advantage of the necessary relaxation of the former and, rebounding, like the stone of Sysyphus, recovers its lost ground and renews the toil of its more powerful opponent. Breathing is in a great measure the effect of this interminable contest between the elasticity of the lungs and the irritability of the diaphragm.[5]

Carson returned to the subject in a later paper entitled *On Lesions of the Lung* which he presented to the Literary and Philosophical Society of Liverpool in November 1821. After stating his belief that the difficulty observed in the healing of parenchymal lesions of the lung was due to this elasticity, which kept the lung permanently on the stretch, he suggested that if the organ were reduced to a state of collapse then the difficulty would be overcome.

> For in this stage the diseased part would be placed in a quiescent state, receiving little or no disturbance from the movements of respiration which would be performed solely by the other lung, and the divided surfaces would be brought into close contact by the same resilient power which before had kept them asunder. A wound or abscess in this lung, would be placed in circumstances at least as favourable to the healing process, as the same affection in any other part of the body.

He told of his experimental work on this theme and how, when he had induced artificial pneumothorax in rabbits, the animals quickly recovered. He then proceeded:

> It not infrequently and in the early stages perhaps generally happens, that the deplorable disease termed consumption has its seat in one lung

5   Carson, J. (1822) *Essays, Physiological and Practical*. p. 23. Liverpool: F. B. Wright.

only . . . The means we possess of reducing this lung to a state of collapse, or of divesting it for a time of its peculiar functions are equally simple and safe.[6]

He mentioned the need to collapse the lung gradually 'by admitting a small quantity of air into the cavity of the chest at one time, and allowing an interval to exist between the successive admissions' and he even spoke of the possibility of establishing pneumothorax successively on both sides for the management of bilateral disease. He concluded his address with these prophetic paragraphs, presented with a modesty which only serves to enhance the stature of the man:

> The experience of every age and country too well attests the insignificancy of all our efforts to arrest even for a moment the slow but steadily onward pace of this fatal malady; and if any addition to the proof of its incurability under every method of treatment hitherto proposed were required, that addition would be supplied by the views, supposing them to be just, that have been exhibited of its nature . . . It has long been my opinion that if ever this disease is to be cured, and it is an event of which I am by no means disposed to despair, it must be accomplished by mechanical means, or in other words by a surgical operation. Whether the method proposed will be found practicable, or, if practicable, to the desired extent beneficial, or whether, as will be supposed by far most probable, it may amuse for a moment then like all its predecessors sink into deserved neglect, are questions which must be left to the decision of time. Whatever may be the event, I shall have this consolation, that I incur no risk in this case by any proposition that may be made, of diverting the current of enquiry into a channel that shall be less productive than any of those in which it has hitherto run.[7]

Carson had the courage of his convictions and put his ideas to clinical trial in two cases. The attendant surgeon made incisions between the sixth and seventh ribs of each patient, calculated to admit air freely into the chest[8] but in neither case was collapse of the lung obtained due to widespread pleural adhesions. There is no evidence that Carson pursued the matter further and one is thus left to reflect on how he might have proceeded had a free pleural space been found. He was quite definite in his view that the production of lung collapse should be 'by degrees only' which suggests that he must have envisaged the possibility of serial thoracic wall incisions, a programme

6 *Ibid.* pp. 58–9.
7 *Ibid.* pp. 64–5.
8 Brown, L. (3) p. 239.

which would have demanded considerable fortitude from his patients. It is probable that Carson, with his ingenious ideas and sound grasp of physiological principles, would have found the solution to this difficulty but it is also certain that, in the pre-Listerian era in which he practised, he would in the process have created as great a problem as that which he was setting out to solve. Nevertheless the credit for the first scientifically based enunciation of the principles of collapse therapy rightly belongs to this Liverpool physician who anticipated Forlanini by nearly 60 years.

Carson's merits were recognized and honoured by his contemporaries in his election to the Fellowship of the Royal Society in 1837 but his work was ill-understood and conveniently forgotten by his successors. In the end justice was done, for in 1909 Carson's papers were triumphantly resuscitated by S. Daus[9] and his name was rightly added to the list of those who have made major contributions to the history of tuberculosis.

During the interval between Carson's publications and the first paper by Forlanini a very few sporadic references to the possibilities of therapeutic lung collapse appeared in the literature. In America in 1835 Daniel McRuer of Bangor, Maine, a Scot and a graduate of Edinburgh, who had reached the United States by way of a shipwreck and had found the country to his liking, put forward the idea of artificial pneumothorax in a communication to the *Boston Medical and Surgical Journal*.[10] He based his argument on the principle that rest was one of the best remedial measures being indispensable when reunion of a part was to be effected and then he posed the question:

> Will we not be justified to suspend the action of a diseased lung, by puncturing the chest, under the following restrictions. When the disease is confined to one lung; when pleuritis is not present; when there is still remaining stamina sufficient to enable the system to recover?

Unfortunately he elected to illustrate his thesis with the case history of a nine-year-old girl who, after an acute respiratory infection 'developed symptoms of confirmed phthisis'. The subsequent course of the illness makes it clear that it was, in fact, a post-pneumonic empyema which responded to intercostal drainage but in spite of this piece of clinical irrelevance one must recognize that the idea of

9 Daus, S. (1909) Historisches und Kritisches über künstlichen Pneumothorax bei Lungenschwindsucht. *Therapie Gegenw. 1*, 221, 277.
10 McRuer, D. (1835) Consumption. *Boston. med. surg. J. 12*, 10.

artificial pneumothorax had occurred to McRuer, he had put it in writing and consequently he is deserving of his place in the historical record.

Another name mentioned as an early proponent of this method of treatment is that of Francis Hopkins Ramadge but the claims which have been made on his behalf do not stand up to critical scrutiny. An Irish physician practising in London, he had attracted adverse publicity by his unwise defence of an unqualified practitioner and his subsequent libel action against the *Lancet*.[11] Nevertheless ostracism by many of his colleagues did not deter him from proceeding with the publication of his book *Consumption Curable; and the Manner in which Nature as well as Remedial Art operates in Effecting a Healing Process; explained and illustrated by numerous remarkable and interesting cases.* Following a preface in which he names three of the leading physicians of the day and enlarges on their incompetence, he then gives his own views on treatment:

> After the careful examination of at least three thousand dead bodies, and after having had under my care many thousand consumptive cases, my fixed opinion is, that ulcers of the lung are more effectually cured, and a fresh formation of tubercles prevented, by an expansion of the vesicular structures of the lung.

He elaborates on this theme later:

> I never knew a consumptive person who did not lose all his formidable symptoms and regain health, when an emphysematous, or a semi-asthmatic change had early taken place; and, likewise, I never knew an individual to become consumptive who was subject to chronic catarrh, or to any species of asthma.[12]

The treatment which he proposed was designed 'to effect pulmonary expansion by some artificial means' and the artificial means involved 'inhaling, performed two or three times daily, for half an hour each time'. The inhaling was, in effect, forced respiration through a narrow bore tube and Ramadge recommended its continuance for six months or longer believing firmly that it brought about emphysematous changes which, by increasing the volume of the lung, forced the walls

---

11   Dr Ramadge's actions for Libel (1832) *Lond. med. surg. J.* 212.
12   Ramadge, F. H. (1836) *Consumption Curable; and the Manner in which Nature as well as Remedial Art operates in effecting a Healing Process; explained and illustrated by numerous remarkable and interesting cases.* 3rd ed. p. 34. London: Longman.

of tuberculous cavities into contact and eventually union. His confidence was unbounded:

'I have never known inhalation fail when resorted to in the incipient stage of consumption, and am firmly of the opinion that when pursued under the eye of a skilful practitioner . . . it never will.'[13]

It is probable that the legend of an association between Ramadge and the idea of artificial pneumothorax had its origin in two or three of the voluminous case histories with which he embellished the appendix to his volume under such headings as *Supposed Consumption cured by Paracentesis*, or, more simply, *Consumption cured by Paracentesis*. The first of these was almost certainly a case of empyema with a bronchopleural fistula while the remaining two appear to have been large tuberculous cavities which were deliberately punctured with a trocar 'to ensure the emission of the air and thus effect a diminution of the cavity by the expansion of the inferior lobe'.[14] Ramadge's ideas were indeed far removed from those put forward so modestly and thoughtfully by James Carson and there is nothing in his book which offers even a vestige of support for the continued inclusion of his name amongst the precursors of Forlanini.

While Carson's views and proposals had been based on physiological considerations the next evidence of a changing outlook came as the result of clinical observation. Up until the early part of the nineteenth century the occurrence of a spontaneous pneumothorax as a complication of phthisis had been regarded as providing an inevitably fatal combination. This accepted piece of clinical dogma was now to be challenged by some of the leading clinicians of the day. In 1832 James Houghton reported improvement in a case of advanced phthisis as the result of a spontaneous pneumothorax,[15] while in 1837 William Stokes wrote

that in many cases where the disease (pneumothorax) becomes chronic, we may observe a singular suspension of the usual symptoms of phthisis. The phthisical countenance disappears; the sweats cease; the pulse I have known in some cases to become quiet, and the patient may gain flesh and strength to a surprising degree.[16]

13 *Ibid.* p. 100.
14 *Ibid.* p. 156.
15 Houghton, J. (1832) Account of a remarkable case of pneumothorax. *Dubl. J. med. Sci. 1*, 313.
16 Stokes, W. (1837) *A Treatise on the Diagnosis and Treatment of Diseases of the Chest.* Part I, p. 531. Dublin: Hodges & Smith.

Similar observations were later made by Hérard who, in 1881, presented details of two cases to the French Congress at Algiers in which recorded symptomatic improvement was shown at autopsy to have been accompanied by evidence of local improvement in cavitated lung lesions.[17]

In 1885 William Cayley induced an artificial pneumothorax by open incision of the chest wall to control a severe haemoptysis in a case of phthisis.[18] The bleeding ceased and, although the patient died a few days later from disseminated tuberculosis, there had been no recurrence of the haemorrhage. When he reported the case at the Clinical Society of London it aroused much interest, provoking a lively and intelligent discussion which led Rist to comment at a much later date that, if Cayley had invented a flawless and efficient technique, collapse therapy would probably have progressed more rapidly and against considerably less opposition than it was eventually to encounter.

The great Potain had by now become interested in the problem, again as the result of his own clinical observations, and, being convinced that collapse of the lung was beneficial because it immobilized the organ, he very reasonably argued that re-expansion, since it would terminate the immobilization, and thus stimulate afresh the underlying lesions, should not be permitted. He translated his theory into practice in three cases, complicated by spontaneous pneumothorax with an accompanying effusion, in which he aspirated the fluid and injected sterilized air.[19] One of these three patients, a case of bilateral phthisis, died after showing some temporary improvement. The other two made good recoveries; one of them, a man in whose sputum tubercle bacilli had been demonstrated (a very new test at that period) had become sputum-negative at the end of his treatment which is recorded as having lasted 288 days during which time he had had three air injections.

In spite of Potain's prestige and authority this aspect of his work was greeted with utter indifference. He had, however, stimulated one of his pupils, Toussaint, into studying more closely the question of

17 Herard, A. (1882) Quoted by Rist, E. (1912–13) Communication au Associat. Francais pour l'Avancement des Sciences. *Q. Jl Med. i,* 259.
18 Cayley, W. (1885) A case of haemoptysis treated by the induction of pneumothorax so as to collapse the lung. *Trans. clin. Soc. Lond. 18.* 278.
19 Potain, C. (1888) Des injections intrapleurales d'air sterilisé dans le traitement des epanchements pleuraux consécutifs au pneumothorax. *Bull. Acad. Méd. 19,* 537.

spontaneous pneumothorax in phthisis upon which subject, after collecting 24 cases, he wrote his thesis.[20] In this he concluded that the complication of pneumothorax, particularly if it occurred early in the course of phthisis, was not so serious as had been taught; but, while he had been impressed by this finding, he still found himself unable to support wholeheartedly those who advised surgical intervention as a therapeutic measure.

Inconclusive as Toussaint's work may have appeared it is believed to have influenced one man who had already thought long and deeply about the whole question of spontaneous pneumothorax and about the possibility of making remedial use of artificial pneumothorax in tuberculosis. Carlo Forlanini was born in Milan in 1847. He interrupted his medical studies to serve with Garibaldi in 1866 but eventually graduated at the University of Pavia in 1870. His early appointments were at the Ospedale Maggiore of Milan where he remained until 1884 when he was appointed professor of physical diagnosis at Turin, returning ultimately to his old university of Pavia as professor of clinical medicine. His interest in tuberculosis became apparent at an early stage in his career when at a hospital staff meeting in 1874 he presented a paper on *A case of tuberculosis of the myocardium with large nodes*. His subsequent publications indicated that this interest was maintained and it led him eventually to the first of his historic communications on the therapy of tuberculosis when he published, in August 1882, his long paper *As a contribution to the surgical therapy of phthisis. Ablation of the lung? Artificial pneumothorax?*[21] In this study he referred initially to some German experimental work on extirpation of the lung which had left him unconvinced: 'It does not seem to me that, at least for the present, we can think seriously of partial or total ablation of the lung.' After citing the work of Toussaint and after a detailed analysis of the clinical notes of Hérard and Meusnier he set out his own considered view.

> That they would tend to establish that an infectious and contagious disease is immediately interrupted in its course; the micro-organisms that alone sustain it, that are its essence, are rendered impotent, killed by the sudden onset of a condition of an essentially and purely mechanical and accidental nature.

20 Toussaint, E. (1880) Sur la marche de la tuberculisation pulmonaire. Influence du pneumothorax. *Thèse de Paris*.
21 Lojacono, S. (1934) Forlanini's original communication on artificial pneumothorax. *Tubercle*. p. 54.

Forlanini then went on to put his proposition that

> If a spontaneous pneumothorax arrests, as such, the course of phthisis in
> a lung, why should we not cause in a consumptive an artificial pneumo-
> thorax through the chest wall with the necessary precautions that will be
> useful in preventing secondary pleuritic processes? ... As for me not
> only am I persuaded that actually the pneumothorax was the only and
> essential reason for the change in the course of phthisis, but for some
> time I have been convinced, *a priori*, of the beneficial influence that,
> given certain conditions, pneumothorax *must* exert on the phthisiogenic
> process of the lung; and for my part the cases of Toussaint, Hérard and
> Meusnier were not a revelation, but only the confirmation and perhaps
> the practical proof of the justification of a firm conviction already
> acquired.

He explained that 'the lung ... becomes consumptive because,
differently from all the other viscera, it is in an unceasing motion of
expansion and reduction' from which he deduced that

> the phthisiogenic process must terminate in the lung which is im-
> mobilized by pneumothorax. And this is how the full agreement between
> what I shall call 'my point of view' in phthisis, to which I had already
> come with the aforesaid reasoning, and the clinical facts of Toussaint,
> Hérard and Meusnier, that I learnt later, make the proposition of inducing
> artificial pneumothorax in consumptives appear reasonable to me.

In elaborating further on his proposition Forlanini made it clear that
the pneumothorax should be of such a degree as to immobilize the
lung thus suppressing its movement and, in his view, thereby making
the procedure equivalent to total ablation, but he did stress the need
to ensure that the function of the healthier lung was not disturbed
advising that 'the volume of gas and its pressure be such as not to
displace the mediastinum'. He considered that artificial pneumothorax would have two major advantages over ablation of the lung in
'the ease of execution and the relative harmlessness of the procedure,
and the possibility that the function of the operated lung be regained
entirely or in part'. He concluded his communication thus:

> It has, to my mind, requisites worthy of consideration. It would cer-
> tainly seem rash to me to-day to attempt it directly on a consumptive.
> But when by experimentation on animals it will be demonstrated that the
> physician can quantify with precision artificial pneumothorax and
> always control its volume, and the absolute harmlessness of proper gases,

brought into contact with the pleura, will also have been demonstrated, then this operative procedure should seem logical and legitimate.

This somewhat verbose publication, based entirely on theory and without any supporting experimental evidence, not unnaturally failed to arouse interest or excite comment but Forlanini was not deterred and over the succeeding 12 years he proceeded very slowly and cautiously with the problem of translating theory into practice. He returned to the subject of artificial pneumothorax on the occasion of the Eleventh International Medical Congress at Rome in 1894, armed on this occasion with some clinical facts.[22] After he had discussed the case histories of two patients whom he believed to have been cured of their phthisis by the intervention of a spontaneous pneumothorax, he stated that he had induced artificial pneumothorax in a certain number of tuberculosis patients in whom the extent, gravity and bilateral distribution of the lesions might be held to have removed any reasonable hope.

> My purpose could not be more than that of studying the tolerance of the patient for the pneumothorax induced systematically, and the best operative technique. In short, to prepare the soil for the future.

He concluded by giving details of his technique in which he employed a large hypodermic needle and used nitrogen rather than air as a filling medium.

At the beginning of treatment Forlanini gave small amounts of the gas (200 to 250 cc) daily, then every other day, ultimately extending the interval to one week or longer. He was satisfied that the pleura tolerated the gas well and, while he did not detect any consequent effusion, he did notice that the rate of absorption of the gas by the pleura gradually slowed down. He commented also on the frequency with which pleural adhesions interfered with the degree of collapse thus diminishing its therapeutic value, a finding which in this instance must have been considerably exaggerated by the nature of his clinical material. As a direct consequence of utilizing such advanced cases his results were extremely poor, as indeed he had anticipated; but he did feel that the main objective of the exercise, to establish the safety of the method, had been attained and that its trial in more promising clinical material could now be justified.

22 Forlanini, C. (1894) Primo tentativi di pneumotorace artificiale della tisi pulmonare. *Gazz. med. Torino* *45*, 381.

He delayed no longer in putting his contention to test and his next paper, in 1895, reported the result of an artificial pneumothorax in a 17-year-old girl described as having fever, emaciation, abundant purulent sputum laden with tubercle bacilli, and cavitated disease in the right upper lobe. A pneumothorax was induced in October 1894 and by February 1895 not only was the patient's condition greatly improved in all respects but the sputum had become scanty in amount and negative on direct smear examination. This progress had been maintained and, after she had been sent for a mountain holiday in July 1895, she returned to work, being given refills of nitrogen at six-weekly intervals.[23]

Even after this communication Forlanini's work aroused little interest in his own country and none at all abroad. No one, even in Italy, felt sufficiently stimulated to explore the matter further and, although continuing to work quietly on the subject in his own clinic, he retreated behind a barrier of public silence. This silence was maintained until 1906 when he published, this time in a German journal, an account of 25 cases which he had treated since 1895 and, in presenting these, he claimed the right of priority in the invention of artificial pneumothorax.[24]

The staking of such a claim for priority had become necessary since, during the years of his self-imposed silence, a formidable rival had appeared in the United States. John Benjamin Murphy who was born at Appleton, Wisconsin, in 1857, graduated in medicine from Rush College and spent the succeeding two years in postgraduate study in various centres, including Vienna, A man of powerful personality, extraordinary energy and much ability, all conveniently allied to a useful flair for publicity, he quickly made a name for himself in his own country. He was interested in many fields of surgery, but it so happened that when he was invited to deliver the Oration on Surgery at the meeting of the American Medical Association in 1898 he chose to speak on *Surgery of the Lung*.[25] In the course of this oration which touched on many aspects of lung surgery, he devoted some time to the subject of pulmonary tuberculosis.

> Tuberculosis of the lung has been considered a medical and not a surgical disease. In a few instances the surgeon has had the courage to open

23 Forlanini, C. (1895) Primo caso di tisi pulmonare monolaterale avanzata curato felicimente col pneumotorace artificiale. *Gazz. med. Torino 46*, 857.
24 Forlanini, C. (1906) Zur Behandlung der Lungenschwindsucht durch kunstlich erzeugten Pneumothorax. *Dt med. Wschr. 32*, 1401.
25 Murphy, J. B. (1898) Surgery of the Lung. *J. Am. med. Ass. 31*, 151, 208, 281.

and drain cavities in the lung . . . With these few exceptions, the disease has been left entirely to the care of the physicians. We ask ourselves, what has been achieved in tuberculosis? With the exception of a thorough knowledge of its etiology and pathology, comparatively nothing . . . From a therapeutic standpoint, we had hoped and still hope, that tuberculosis may be cured, alleviated or curtailed in its destructive effects by products derived by the tubercular bacillus under certain conditions. The results barely justify a continuation of that hope. Can surgery contribute anything toward the repair of tubercular lesions of the lung?

After this hard-hitting opening Murphy went on to explain how he had arrived at the idea of producing collapse of the tuberculous lung and in mustering his arguments he was really reiterating the principles so clearly set out by Carson many years before.

The pathology of repair of pulmonary tubercular cavities involves certain physical conditions which are peculiar to the chest . . . namely the constant resistance of the bony framework against contraction, the effort of expansion of the cavity in each respiratory act. The best illustrations exist in large empyemic cavities . . . Allow the wall of the abscess to collapse, to empty thoroughly, and it will heal as other abscesses of the same pathologic character; this, I believe, is the keynote to the successful treatment of pulmonary cavities. How to overcome this resistance of the chest wall was a stimulus to my investigations in lung surgery, and led to the hope that not only might pulmonary cavities be obliterated by permitting or forcing their collapse, but that primary tuberculosis might be encapsulated by mechanical immobilization of the diseased portion by collapse and enforced rest of the lung as a respiratory apparatus, thus allowing the cicatrization and encapsulation of the tubercular foci; in other words, that tuberculosis of the lung might be treated as we treat tuberculosis of the joints, by immobilizing and enforcing physiologic rest . . . The methods of obtaining pulmonary quiesence or collapse are: (1) by permitting or forcing collapse of the lung by separation of the parietal pleura and intrathoracic compression (extrapleural pneumothorax); (2) by removing the bony resistance and allowing collapse of the chest wall, thus favouring contraction and cicatrization (thoracoplasty); (3) allowing the lung to collapse by intrapleural injection of gas or fluid. The third method appears to offer more than any others.

Having formulated a theory Murphy was not one to waste time over submitting it to the test of practical experience. He devised a simple apparatus of movable bottles attached to a trocar, worked out a simple, though by later standards a dangerous technique and went ahead. At induction he gave an enormous quantity of nitrogen, varying from 1155 to 3300 cc gauging the exact amount by his assessment of the patient's distress and dyspnoea and the degree of displacement of the mediastinum and diaphragm. At the time of his communication to the American Medical Association he had attempted pneumothorax in seven cases. In two the attempt had failed, due to pleural adherence, but in the remaining five the results were claimed to be excellent, although it is necessary to mention that the case-histories were scanty and the follow-up minimal, while in only one instance had a refill been given. Such evidence seems barely sufficient to justify Murphy's somewhat extravagant claim. Probably his greatest contribution, and the one which was least appreciated, was his emphasis on the value of radiology in the control of pneumothorax therapy for, although it was only three years since Röntgen's discovery, Murphy was illustrating his remarks with X-ray plates showing the lung collapse. He considered that these indicated a very slow absorption of the gas and, since he had visualized the treatment as lasting no longer than three to six months at most, one has here the explanation of why only a single refill had been given.

This oration by the master surgeon aroused great interest and hope throughout America, bringing him an avalanche of letters from patients with tuberculosis. He had to make a choice between the practice of surgery or of pulmonary tuberculosis and he unhesitatingly chose surgery, being aided in his selection by the fact that he had already decided that the whole question of pneumothorax therapy was so simple and straightforward that it could be safely left in the hands of the physicians! He never collapsed another lung and turned the work over to one of the assistants in his private practice, August Lemke. Lemke reported a series of cases in 1899,[26] claiming good results, but again assessment has been made difficult by lack of detail in the case histories and by the brevity of the follow-up. It shortly became clear, however, that interest in artificial pneumothorax in the United States, initially stimulated by the magic of the Murphy name, was still only a feeble flame and even that flickered to extinction with Lemke's death in 1906 when, for a few years, the practice of pneumothorax therapy virtually ceased throughout America.

But the work of Murphy and Lemke had not been in vain for they

26 Lemke, A. F. (1899) Report of cases of pulmonary tuberculosis treated with intrapleural injections of nitrogen, with a consideration of the pathology of compression of the tuberculous lung. *J. Am. med. Ass.* *33*, 959, 1023, 1077.

succeeded, where Forlanini had so far failed, in arousing interest in the
idea in Europe. The reason for this success can almost certainly be
ascribed to the difference in the wares which the rivals were offering.
Murphy was selling a surgical cure for tuberculosis, a cure to be
achieved by one or two treatments only and this appeared an attractive
package if one ignored the fact that the work was based on but a few
months experience. Forlanini, on the other hand, was promoting a
long-term programme of lung compression necessitating frequent
treatments over a period of years and offering no guarantee of ultimate
success. Murphy's confident predictions struck a spark where
Forlanini's caution had failed to ignite and Ludolph Brauer of
Marburg reported his first case of artificial pneumothorax 'nach
Murphy' in the *Aerztlicher Verein* at Marburg in 1905 followed by a
second in 1906.[27] In this latter the clinical details were set out with
great care and thoroughness, and, at the time of reporting, four refills
had been given with much benefit to the patient. In devising his technique Brauer stressed the importance to the operator of knowing the
exact position of his needle point before permitting gas to flow: in
order to ensure this he cut down on the pleura and introduced the
needle under direct vision—a procedure that he was later happy to
abandon with the advent of the water manometer.

It seems probable that Forlanini was galvanized into the publication
of his 25 cases by Brauer's paper, which had hailed Murphy as the
originator of the method. The same spur may have decided him to
publish in Germany rather than in the Italy which had earlier failed to
appreciate his work. In both decisions he was fully justified for, by
general agreement thereafter, Forlanini has passed into history as the
creator of artificial pneumothorax therapy but, in awarding the
laurels to the Italian it is only right and just that homage should be paid
to the memory of James Carson of Liverpool and the birth of the idea.

The publication of Murphy and Lemke had been studied by a
notable Danish physician, Christian Saugman, who, using their technique, induced pneumothorax in two or three cases but without any
notable success. In 1906 he read Forlanini's German paper and
immediately ordered the apparatus. This action by Saugman was to
mark yet another milestone on the path of progress for he saw at once
the danger involved in Forlanini's method, in which the pleura was
punctured with a hollow needle in permanent communication with a

27 Brauer, L. (1906) Die Behandlung der einseitigen Lungenphthisis mit kunstlichen
Pneumothorax (nach Murphy). *Munch. med. Wschr. 53*, 337.

cylinder containing nitrogen under positive pressure. This meant in practice that he only knew that his needle point was in the pleural space when the gas flowed freely—a blind and dangerous method which explained the many incidents of 'pleural eclampsy' encountered by Forlanini. These were undoubtedly episodes of minute gas embolism, and, although this explanation was always strongly resisted by the Italian, it constituted a risk which Saugman was not prepared to take. He made his own contribution to the history of artificial pneumothorax by adding to the apparatus a water manometer which permitted measurement of the gas pressure within the needle.[28] This information, by indicating to the operator when the needle point was between the pleural surfaces, added immeasurably to the safety of both induction and of refills.

During the period 1906 to 1908 other European centres became alert to the possibilities of this method of treatment and cautious exploration of its potential was begun by workers in Germany, Denmark, Norway and Switzerland—all with varying results and consequently varying opinions. Dumarest, who had studied at Forlanini's clinic, was the first to introduce the method into France[29] followed quickly by G. Küss of Agincourt who· reported his first three cases in 1910 when he also described his ingenious apparatus.[30] Edouard Rist of the Laënnec Hospital in Paris, having been much impressed by Küss, began to employ artificial pneumothorax in 1911 and two years later published in English a most excellent review of the whole subject.[31]

In 1909 the post-Lemke hiatus in the United States came to a close with a revival of interest in pneumothorax therapy led by Mary Lapham[32] and by Robinson and Cleaveland Floyd.[33] The latter two not only established the use of pneumothorax in Boston but, by the many demonstrations which they carried out in different centres,

28 Brown, L. (3) p. 272.
29 Dumarest, F. (1909) Du pneumothorax chirurgical dans le traitement de la phthisie pulmonaire. *Bull. Med.* February.
30 Küss, G. (1910) La technique et les résultates immédiates du pneumothorax artificiel dans les formes avancées unilatérales de la tuberculose pulmonaire. *Bull. Mém. Soc. Méd. Paris 2*, 88.
31 Rist, E. (1912–13) Artificial Pneumothorax: A critical review. *Q. Jl Med. 1*, 259.
32 Lapham, M. E. (1911) The treatment of pulmonary tuberculosis by artificial pneumothorax. *Sth. med. J. 4*, 742.
33 Robinson, S. & Floyd, C.(1912) Artificial pneumothorax as a treatment of pulmonary tuberculosis. *Archs intern. Med. 9*, 452.

contributed largely to the extension of the method throughout America.

Artificial pneumothorax was introduced into Britain, the land of Carson and of Cayley, by Claude Lillingston who, himself ill with tuberculosis, had had a pneumothorax established at Mesnalien sanatorium in Norway. He returned to Britain to work at Mundesley Sanatorium with Vere Pearson who recorded that Lillingston, with the assistance of his wife, gave himself his first refill in England. Pearson gave the second refill after which he and Lillingston, aided by the sanatorium carpenter, designed a safe and effective apparatus which was to be widely used throughout the country in the years ahead. From Mundesley the gospel of pneumothorax spread outwards, Lillingston and Pearson in their turn initiating such early British workers as Clive Rivière, Burton-Fanning and Woodcock.[34]

The recognition of Forlanini as the High Priest of the new treatment implied acceptance of his view that the full benefits of collapse therapy could only be obtained when the lung had been kept in a condition of complete immobility for a prolonged period. The first to challenge this doctrine was Maurizio Ascoli who, in 1912, pointed out that mere relaxation of the lung was quite as effective as the compression favoured by the Master.[35] He found that such relaxation could be obtained with intrapleural pressures less than atmospheric, a finding which led him to suggest—and to put into practice—simultaneous bilateral artificial pneumothorax, thus bringing about a significant extension of the range of the treatment. A similar idea occurred independently to W. Parry Morgan who in 1913 noted that, if only a small amount of gas was introduced into the pleural space, it tended to accumulate over the diseased areas. The result was that when inspiration took place

> those portions of the lung which remained normally expansible will dilate and tend to come into contact with the chest wall, while the displaced gas will find lodgment over the less expansible portions, and prevent the increase in the elastic tension which would be produced if the gas were not present.[36]

34 Pearson, S. V. (1946) *Men, Medicine and Myself.* p. 95. London: Museum Press.
35 Ascoli, M. (1912) Ueber den künstlichen Pneumothorax nach Forlanini. *Dt. med. Wschr. 38*, 1782.
36 Morgan, W. P. (1913) On the possibility of achieving by partial pneumothorax the advantages of complete pneumothorax. *Lancet 2*, 18.

This was the basis of 'selective collapse' of which much was to be heard thereafter and Morgan himself reverted to the subject remarking that

> The effect of the introduction into the pleural cavity of a quantity of gas sufficient to produce only a partial collapse is a considerable limitation of movement of the diseased parts and, what is more important, the prevention of that pumping action which would otherwise produce auto-inoculation; that is, we obtain by means of a partial collapse the same advantages as by complete, and we should expect the same result.[37]

Like Ascoli, Morgan appreciated that both lungs could be treated at one and the same time and he became the first in Britain to practice simultaneous bilateral pneumothorax.

The exploratory work on therapeutic pneumothorax which was taking place during the first decade of the twentieth century soon rivetted attention on the high incidence of pleural adhesions and the extent to which these could interfere with efficient lung collapse. Carson had already established that pleural adherence could obliterate the pleural space completely, making pneumothorax impossible. This was later to be confirmed by others in larger numbers and in greater detail. Saugman[38] reported that in his series of cases which he had judged suitable for a trial of pneumothorax, 11 per cent showed completely adherent pleurae. Hamman and Sloan,[39] from the Johns Hopkins hospital in Baltimore, had 15 per cent totally adherent while Burrell[40] from the Brompton Hospital and Rivière[41] from the London Chest Hospital had figures of 12.7 per cent and 20 per cent respectively. There was, therefore, an appreciable proportion of patients in whom pneumothorax was therapeutically desirable but technically impossible. Thereafter came those, relatively small in number, whose pleural space was completely adhesion-free and who presented few problems followed by a much larger group in whom a pneumothorax could be successfully induced but where a partial degree of adherence,

37 Morgan, W. P. (1917) Artificial pneumothorax in the treatment of pulmonary tuberculosis. *Q. Jl Med. ii,* 1.
38 Saugman, C. (1914) Zur Technik des künstlichen Pneumothorax. *Beitr. Klin Tuberk. 31,* 571.
39 Hamman, L. & Sloan, M. F. (1913) Induced pneumothorax in the treatment of pulmonary disease. *Johns Hopkins Hosp. Bull. 24,* 53.
40 Burrell, L. S. T. & Macnalty, A. S. (1922) Report on artificial pneumothorax in *Med. Res. Council Special Report Series.* No. 67.
41 Rivière, C. (1919) The pneumothorax treatment of pulmonary tuberculosis. *Tubercle i.* 114.

with the adhesions usually located over the site of the lesion, prevented satisfactory pulmonary relaxation.

It was clear that total pleural adherence required a new approach and procedures to cope with this contingency were already being explored and will be described later. Partial pleural adherence on the other hand appeared to offer some scope for a possible local solution. The first attempt at such a local solution was made by Friedrich of Marburg in 1908[42] when he proposed and carried out an operation which involved opening the chest and pleural cavity and dividing the adhesions under direct vision. The results reported by Friedrich, and by a number of other surgeons who adopted his method, were poor; there was a high incidence of serious or fatal operative and post-operative complications and the method was hastily abandoned.

A more ingenious and acceptable approach was devised by Hans Christian Jacobaeus of Stockholm who had become interested in the diagnostic possibilities of endoscopy, both of the pleural and peritoneal cavities, and in pursuit of this interest had invented the thoracoscope. He was now to find an additional use for this instrument.

> By thoracoscopy in the pneumothorax treatment of lung tuberculosis an especially fine picture of cord or membrane-like adhesions between lung and thoracic wall is obtained. This led me to try to work out a method under the guidance of the thoracoscope of removing such adhesions as impede treatment.

After quoting figures published by Gravesen from Vejlefjord sanatorium which showed clearly the vastly different prognosis of the patient with a complete and adhesion-free pneumothorax as compared with his less fortunate fellow in whom adhesions prevented such a satisfactory collapse, he continued:

> As it was rather easy to observe the above adhesions by thoracoscopy the idea occurred of cauterizing them by introducing a galvanocautery through another opening under the guidance of the thoracoscope. My first attempt was made in 1913, and since then I have performed, altogether, seventy-five such operations.[43]

42 Friedrich, P. L. (1908) The operative treatment of unilateral lung tuberculosis by total mobilization of the chest wall by means of thoraco-plastic pleuro-pneumolysis. *Surgery. Gynec. Obstet. 7,* 632.
43 Jacobaeus, H. C. (1922–23) The cauterization of adhesions in artificial pneumothorax treatment of pulmonary tuberculosis under thoracoscopic control. *Proc. Roy. Soc. Med.* 45.

He considered that in 50 of these 75 he had obtained a good clinical result. Similar figures were soon being reported by his Scandinavian colleagues who quickly realized the value of the procedure and lost no time in adopting it in their own sanatoria and clinics.

From Scandinavia thoracoscopy and adhesion section, later to be termed closed intrapleural pneumonolysis, spread steadily throughout Europe and America until it eventually came to be accepted as an indispensable adjunct to the proper practice of pneumothorax therapy. Individual operators from time to time made modifications in equipment and in technique but these were minor changes only and throughout the operation remained essentially the same as that devised by Hans Christian Jacobaeus who is rightly credited with this major advance and whose name may properly be set alongside that of Forlanini—the two great practical innovators in this field.

Although the development of artificial pneumothorax treatment had rested mainly in the hands of the physicians the surgeons had by no means relinquished their claims to a stake in the therapy of phthisis. Devout believers in the radical approach, their interest was first directed towards the possibility of resection of the diseased area. There was ample evidence from numerous animal experiments, particularly those by Glück, to show that removal of a lung or lobe could be done with relative safety[44] while in 1882 Block, after a further series of experiments both on healthy animals and on others which had been infected with tuberculous sputum, reported successful resection results with frequent survival and apparent cure. Walton, who had been present at a demonstration of these results by Block, wrote a letter to the *Boston Medical and Surgical Journal* saying:

> The doctor assured us that he had been promised opportunities to operate on the human subject, and that he should do so at an early date, with every hope of successful issue. He found it hard, however, to communicate his unbounded enthusiasm and hopefulness to others, and though much interest was shown in the preparations, many doubts were expressed in the first place as to whether the operation would prove so safe and simple in the human subject as in the rabbit, and in the second place as to whether the operation, if successfully performed, would be as efficacious as anticipated in checking the spread of pulmonary disease.[45]

44   Gluck, T. (1881) Experimenteller Beitrag zur Frage der Lungenextirpation. *Berl. klin. Wschr. 18*, 645.

45   Walton, G. L. (1883) Letter from Berlin: resection of the lung as proposed by Doctor Block. *Boston med. surg. J. 108*, 261.

Undeterred by such scepticism Block allowed his self-confidence to carry him on to disaster. He proceeded to operate on a young woman (said to be related to him) at her urgent request and at a single session he resected both apices. The lungs were said to have been found healthy but the patient died within 24 hours and Block, threatened with legal proceedings, shot himself. In 1885 the Italian surgeon Ruggi, who had also had considerable experience of resection in experimental animals, performed apical resections in two patients.[46] Both died in the immediate post-operative period but the surgeon, unlike Block, did not feel called upon to make any public gesture of dissatisfaction with his results.

The first successful resection for tuberculosis appears to have been accomplished by Tuffier who, in 1891, employing a technique somewhat different from that of his predecessors, removed the right apex in a 19-year-old man.[47] The patient made a satisfactory recovery and is known to have been alive and well four years later. Lowson, in 1893, recorded a rather similar experience,[48] as did Macewen in 1895,[49] but in spite of these isolated successes, resection made little appeal and was abandoned for nearly 40 years while the surgeons turned with energy and enthusiasm to other major, though on the whole less hazardous, operations.

The intital step in this alternative approach appears to have been taken by de Cérenville of Lausanne and in essence it was an attempt to apply the principles enunciated by Carson, although there is no evidence that he was acquainted with Carson's writings. de Cérenville concentrated his attention entirely upon cavities and published an account of his work in 1885.[50] This included four patients, presenting with apical tuberculous cavities, in whom he had resected up to 3.5 cm of the second and third ribs anteriorly in order to break the continuity of the bony thoracic cage in the hope of effecting collapse of the underlying pulmonary cavities. The operations were not attended by any notable success but the idea stimulated others and the

46 Brown, L. (3) p. 285.
47 Tuffier, T. (1892) Résection du sommet du poumon droit pour tuberculose pulmonaire au début; resultat eloignée (18 mos). *Bull. Mém. Soc. Clin. Paris*. N.S. *18*, 726
48 Lowson, D. (1893) A case of pneumonectomy. *Br. med. J. 1*, 1152.
49 Macewen, W. (1906) Some points in the surgery of the lung. *W. Lond. med. J. 11*, 163.
50 de Cerenville, E. B. (1885) De l'intervention operatoire dans les maladies du poumon. *Revue méd. Suisse romande 5*, 141.

years between 1885 and 1906 witnessed a series of minor attacks on the upper ribs by a variety of Continental surgeons.

The next major step was taken by Ludolph Brauer of Marburg. He had noted and been impressed by the results which followed a complete collapse of the lung by pneumothorax and considered that surgeons, if their efforts were to be successful, must aim at attaining a collapse of a comparable degree. He therefore proposed to replace the somewhat timorous nibblings of his colleagues by a massive assault on the thoracic cage, involving the removal of the entire lengths of ribs two to nine inclusive, which he calculated would provide pulmonary compression rather than mere relaxation. The first such operation was performed in 1907 by Paul Leopold Friedrich: the patient, a certain Monsieur Cordier, survived and 14 months later his tuberculosis was reported to be greatly improved.[51] The era of the thoracoplasty operation had arrived and Brauer and Friedrich pressed on. Their subsequent patients were cast in less heroic mould than Monsieur Cordier, three of the first seven dying from the effects of the operation, while a similar high mortality was reported by other surgeons. The surgical shock following the procedure was terrific and when to this was added the hazards of paradoxical respiration and 'mediastinal flutter' then death from acute respiratory insufficiency was just around the corner. A further and very real disadvantage was impairment of the mechanism of cough and sputum in the post-operative phase which led to the retention of secretions and aspiration spread of the disease.

Brauer, convinced of the value of the operation in those who could survive it, endeavoured to evolve a technique which would either eliminate or reduce the major risks. He proposed that the operation be performed in two stages and that smaller lengths of rib be resected; but, even with these modifications, the mortality rate remained unacceptably high and the operation vanished from the surgical scene to be replaced by that proposed by Max Wilms of Heidelberg.[52]

Wilms had been greatly influenced by the experimental work of Boiffin and of Gourdet[53] who, in studying the operative treatment of

51   Alexander, J. (1937) *The Collapse Therapy of Pulmonary Tuberculosis*. p. 27. Springfield, Illinois: C. C. Thomas.

52   Wilms, M. (1912) Eine neue Methode zur Verengerung des Thorax bei Lungen-tuberkulose. *Munch. med. Wschr. 58*, 777.

53   Gourdet, J. (1895) Thoracoplastie postérieure. Étude sur l'aplatissement comparé du thorax par les différents procédés de resection costales. *Inst. int. Biblphie méd. Paris.*

empyema, were able to demonstrate that a much greater reduction in the size of the thoracic cavity occurred when only the paravertebral portions of the ribs were removed. Gourdet, in particular, favoured the removal of the ribs as far back as the transverse processes of the vertebrae. It was left to Wilms to adapt this experimental work to the surgery of pulmonary tuberculosis and to show clearly that rib resections limited to the paravertebral area had a greater healing effect on tuberculous lesions of the lung than any operation yet proposed and that, in addition, this limitation avoided the disastrous post-operative complications encountered by Brauer and Friedrich. Wilm's operation marked such a radical departure from the extensive mutilation of the thoracic cage favoured by Brauer that it was virtually a new procedure. About the same time Ernst Ferdinand Sauerbruch, working independently along the same lines, had produced a some-what similar modification and thus the Wilms–Sauerbruch para-vertebral thoracoplasty came into being. The operation was per-formed in two stages; portions of the lower ribs were resected at the first stage leaving the upper ribs to be dealt with at the second operation.[54] The inclusion of the lower ribs in the resection despite the fact that the disease was generally concentrated in the upper lung field reflected the current belief that rest and relaxation of the whole lung were necessary to secure the best result, while the operative precedence given to the lower stage represented an attempt to avoid the hazards of aspiration spread of infected material from above. Still more modifications were to follow, but before the thoracoplasty operation had emerged in its final shape other examples of surgical ingenuity were to make their appearance on the scene.

Extrapleural pneumonolysis, consisting of the separation of the lung and both pleural layers from the thoracic cage, was first em-ployed by Tuffier in 1893 to control a severe haemoptysis. Later, in 1910, he attempted a more permanent collapse by filling the extra-pleural space with fat taken from the abdominal wall[55] while, in 1913, Baer employed paraffin wax for the same purpose.[56] This procedure, later usually referred to as apicolysis with plombage, played a limited role in treatment for a period of about 15 years after which it was

54   Alexander, J. (50) p. 32.
55   Tuffier, Collapstherapie par décollement pleuro-parietal pour tuberculose au sommet du poumon, greffe d'un fragment de tissue adipeux dans l'espace décollé. *Bull. Mém. Soc. Clin. Paris 49*, 1249.
56   Baer, G. (1913) Ueber extrapleurale Pneumolyse mit sofortiger Plombierung bei lungentuberkulose. *Munch. med. Wschr. 60*, 1587.

almost completely ousted by thoracoplasty. Later, the idea was to be revived in a brief spurt of enthusiasm for the employment of air as a filling medium (extrapleural pneumothorax) and still later there was a temporary renewal of interest when inert substances such as lucite spheres or polythene sponge material were utilized to provide a more permanent form of collapse.

In 1911 a fresh approach was initiated by Stuertz when he suggested that paralysis of one phrenic nerve might afford some collapse of a diseased lower lobe in cases where artificial pneumothroax had failed because of adherent pleurae.[57] Phrenic paralysis proved a popular procedure, not least because of the relative simplicity of its performance, and after considerable changes in technique and in the indications for its use it became firmly established as a basic method of producing a minor, but occasionally valuable, degree of pulmonary relaxation.

Other ideas were put forward such as multiple intercostal nerve paralysis[58] and later scaleniotomy[59] but although ingenious in conception these methods proved ineffective in practice and were rapidly discarded.

Collapse therapy had gained a firm foothold on the therapeutic ladder by 1914 when the outbreak of World War I initiated a startling increase in the incidence of tuberculosis in Europe. This increase, which was both an accompaniment and an aftermath of the war, made imperative the mobilization and exploitation of all possible forms of treatment and ushered in an era in which therapy was dominated by the sanatorium, artificial pneumothorax, phrenic paralysis and thoracoplasty. There had been important developments also in the preventive and public health aspects of the disease which had already been causing serious concern in the closing years of the nineteenth century and which had led to the introduction in Britain of a national tuberculosis scheme on which all future planning, whether preventive or curative, was to be based.

57   Alexander, J. (50) p. 34.
58   Schepelmann, E. (1913) Thierexperimente zur Lungenchirurgie. *Arch. klin. Chir.* *100*, 985.
59   Gale, J. W. & Middleton, W. S. (1931) Scaleniotomy in the surgical treatment of pulmonary tuberculosis. *Archs Surg. 23*, 38.

Chapter Eleven
Tuberculosis and Public Health: A Plan for Prevention

Apart from the legislative steps taken during the eighteenth century by some enlightened communities in southern Europe, there is no evidence that the lack of a programme of prophylaxis against tuberculosis was causing concern elsewhere. This was not due wholly to complete public disinterest—tuberculosis was a killer and was rightly dreaded—but was a reflection of the fatalistic attitude and outlook fostered by the 'anti-contagionists' and the unquestioning acceptance of their view that the disease was transmissible only by heredity. As already indicated in Chapter 5 so ingrained were these ideas that, even after 1882, there was an appreciable time-lag before the full significance of Koch's discovery, and the possibility of preventive action, sank home.

One of the very few to glimpse the opportunity which the identification of the bacillus had opened up was a young Edinburgh physician, Robert Philip, who actually graduated in the year of the discovery. He had intended to make gynaecology his special interest and was studying in Vienna when, on the road to Damascus as it were, he suddenly saw the vision of a vast new field of study, and returned to Edinburgh determined to specialize in tuberculosis. His early efforts met with little encouragement. His seniors made it quite clear that they considered tuberculosis to be an exhausted subject. Everything that was to be known about it was already known and understood and every sensible person realized the hopelessness of even thinking about its prevention and treatment.

In spite of this devastating barrage of disapproval Philip declined to be discouraged; he had surveyed the Edinburgh scene and had concluded that, as far as tuberculosis was concerned, any change could only be a change for the better.

Up until 1887 there was in Edinburgh no central or concerted action in relation to the treatment of pulmonary tuberculosis. Patients were received and excellently treated in the Royal Infirmary and other hospitals, so long as it was possible to keep them. The general dispensaries of the city received and prescribed medically for those consumptive patients who presented themselves for treatment. Such treatment necessarily consisted in the prescription of some form of cough mixture. The duration of the patient's treatment depended on the continuance of the more aggressive symptoms and his faith in the prescriber or prescription. Consumptive patients, when too ill to come to the dispensary, were commonly relegated to the list of chronic or troublesome patients, visited occasionally by a frequently changing series of medical students, whose conceptions of treatment, doubtless excellent as far as they went, did not extend very far.[1]

Philip was convinced of the need for a much more definite and organized effort, a conviction which he succeeded in conveying to others, and in the autumn of 1887,

> having satisfied myself that a well-directed movement towards the end in view would have the approval of those who might take the trouble to think of the matter, I succeeded, with the help of a few kind friends, in establishing the Victoria Dispensary for Consumption in the heart of Edinburgh.

His conception of the scope and functions of a dispensary went far beyond the popular idea of such an institution with its preoccupation with the supply of bottles of free cough mixture to the needy and deserving. He visualized it as the centre to which all poor persons suffering from consumption might be directed in the first instance, and he laid down the routine to be followed:

a The reception and examination of patients at the dispensary and the keeping of a record of everyone thus received, with an account of his illness, history, surroundings and present condition, the record being added to on each subsequent visit.

b The instruction of patients how to treat themselves and how to prevent or minimize the risk of infection to others.

c The dispensing of necessary medicine, disinfectants and sputum bottles, and, where the family conditions warrant it, of foodstuffs and the like.

d The visitation of patients at their own homes, more especially of patients confined to their home or to bed, and this for the purpose of

---

1 Philip, R. W. (1937) *Collected Papers on Tuberculosis*. p. 21. London: Oxford University Press.

treatment and of investigation into the state of the dwelling, the general conditions of life, and the risk of infection to others in the neighbourhood.

e The selection of more likely patients for hospital treatment, either of early cases for sanatoria, or of late cases for some incurable institution.

f The guidance generally of patients, and friends of patients, and other enquirers on questions related to consumption.[2]

These constituted the basic duties and to them he very soon added the systematic examination of family groups, the 'march past' of the contacts.

He believed also that the dispensary had an important part to play in the relief of the financial distress (which so commonly accompanied the disease) by assessing the family income and, where appropriate, putting the household in touch with one or other of the various public or charitable funds. Later he saw yet another activity for the dispensary in

the determination of suitable lines of employment of a light or open-air kind for consumptive patients not requiring hospital treatment. This has been found in my experience one of the most valuable, if sometimes a difficult part, of the Dispensary's operations ... To the care of the Dispensary would naturally return patients who, after sanatorium treatment, remained still on doubtful ground in respect of permanence of cure. These would be similarly advised as to occupation, residence, continuance of treatment, and from time to time would report themselves for fresh examination.[3]

The foundation of the Victoria Dispensary was but the first step in the creation by Philip of the Edinburgh Co-ordinated Scheme of which much more was to be heard in the years to come. The Dispensary became the central point of the organization, the headquarters from which all further operations were planned, with lines of communication connecting it to the other elements in the scheme: the sanatorium, the hospital for advanced cases and, later, the farm colony. From its inception Philip appreciated that for the elaboration and proper maintenance of such a scheme it would be impossible to rely wholly on individual effort or benevolent enterprise. He foresaw and advocated the involvement of the community in the project, acting through the Local Authority, whose executive representative

2 *Ibid.* p. 22.
3 *Ibid.* p. 27.

would be the Medical Officer of Health. The latter would be kept in specially close touch with the dispensary and the hospital for advanced cases and through these he would be enabled to make a considerable contribution to a programme of prevention.

The creation and perfecting of this scheme was Philip's life-work and it became his memorial when, in 1913, the Astor Departmental Committee on Tuberculosis recommended its adoption as the model for a national scheme, a recommendation which secured Government acceptance and gained for Philip a well-deserved knighthood.

During the 20-odd years which intervened between the genesis of the dispensary system and its translation into national policy the brunt of the struggle against tuberculosis was borne by voluntary effort. It had been this type of effort which had led earlier to the foundation of the Brompton Hospital and of the London Chest Hospital and the embers of the fire thus kindled had continued to smoulder. The successful inauguration of the Edinburgh scheme had caused these embers to glow again and finally, fanned by a powerful editorial in *The Practitioner* of June 1898 appealing for 'a national crusade against a national disease',[4] to burst into flame at a memorable meeting held at Marlborough House on 20 December 1898, with the then Prince of Wales presiding. Those attending included leading figures from the main political parties, representatives of the Church, the universities, the world of commerce, and a number of eminent physicians. The object of this heterogeneous gathering was the formation of the National Association for the Prevention of Consumption and other forms of Tuberculosis, a title later changed to that of the National Association for the Prevention of Tuberculosis. The aim of the Association was

> to carry into every dwelling in the land an elementary knowledge of the mode in which consumption is propagated, and of the means by which its spread may be prevented and thus to strengthen the hands of medical men throughout the country who are dealing with individual cases of the disease.[5]

The meeting expressed its support for the methods which the Association proposed to employ namely the instruction of public opinion and the stimulation of popular interest rather than the advocacy of measures of compulsion.

4 Editorial. (June 1898) *Practitioner* p. 568.
5 Williams, H. (1973) *Requiem for a Great Killer*. p. 10 London: Health Horizon.

A committee was formed under the chairmanship of the Earl of Derby, with the Prince of Wales as president, and the new Association got to work. One of its first public acts was the organization of the British Congress on Tuberculosis, which was held in London in 1901 and which proved a resounding success with an attendance of over 3000, including many visitors from abroad, among whom was Robert Koch. A programme of public education began which involved the issuing of numerous pamphlets explaining the facts about tuberculosis in simple terms, the inauguration of lectures and annual conferences and also of exhibitions, including a travelling exhibition which toured far afield in a horse-drawn vehicle. Branches of the parent Association were formed throughout the country, a number of which proceeded to interest themselves in the establishment of dispensaries and sanatoria in their own areas. As a result of this interest 17 sanatoria, owing their inception either directly to the Association or less directly to its influence, were founded.

In Edinburgh the 'few kind friends' with whose help Philip had founded the Victoria Dispensary had evolved into the Royal Victoria Hospital Tuberculosis Trust. While the objectives of the Trust were essentially similar to those of the National Association for the Prevention of Consumption it had one or two additional projects which were peculiarly its own. One was the maintenance of a national sanatorium-colony for Scotland, with facilities for the treatment of all forms of tuberculosis at all ages, which would also serve as a 'live clinical museum' for research and study. The other was to ensure adequate training for future generations of doctors by the foundation of a chair of tuberculosis within the University of Edinburgh. The first of these aims was achieved with the opening of Southfield Sanatorium on the southern outskirts of Edinburgh while the second came to fruition on 16 April 1918 when Sir Robert Philip, the newly appointed professor, delivered his inaugural lecture on *Present Day Outlook on Tuberculosis*.

The year 1909 brought yet another instance of voluntary action with the establishment of the 'Central Fund for the Promotion of the Dispensary System for the Prevention of Tuberculosis' in London. In the same year the first of the city's tuberculosis dispensaries was opened at Paddington to be followed in 1910 by the Marylebone Dispensary.

Thus far the Government had refrained from involving itself seriously with the problem of tuberculosis and indeed Lord Salisbury,

Prime Minister at the time of the formation of the National Association, is on record as saying that he 'deprecated any appeal to legislative interference.' It was, nevertheless, clear to Philip and to many others that, in order to reap the maximum benefit from the dispensary system and to serve adequately the idea of prevention, information about the extent and distribution of tuberculosis in any given district would require to be as complete as possible to enable the administrative machinery to be fully activated.

This meant *notification*; and the very idea of notification constituted a controversial issue. Its opponents argued that, since most of the cases would have been infectious for a prolonged period before notification, much of the damage which the procedure was designed to obviate would already have been done; that, since the tubercle bacillus was known to enjoy a saprophytic existence apart from its human host, measures directed solely to preventing infection from the patient would be ineffective, and that as phthisis was a disease of protracted duration, the carrying out of official preventive measures would be impracticable and if attempted would entail a larger staff than that possessed by any local sanitary authority. Finally there was the inevitable argument about the breach of professional confidence which would be involved in any system of voluntary notification, concerning which Newsholme wrote:

> This is a real difficulty and must necessarily always limit the operation of voluntary notification of phthisis to patients of the poorer classes, and particularly to those treated in connection with the poor law or with public institutions.[6]

A single tentative step along the legislative road had been taken as far back as 1897 with the passing of the Public Health (Scotland) Act which empowered local authorities to do anything in respect of pulmonary tuberculosis which they were entitled to do for any ordinary infectious disease while the Notification Act (Scotland) of 1889 was extended to include pulmonary tuberculosis. A system of voluntary notification was introduced in Edinburgh in 1903 but no further development of significance took place in Scotland until 1906. On 10 March of that year the Scottish Local Government Board issued a circular pronouncing pulmonary tuberculosis to be an infectious disease within the meaning of the Public Health (Scotland)

6   Newsholme, A. (1908) *The Prevention of Tuberculosis.* p. 340 London: Methuen & Co.

Act 1897 and advising that notification was necessary to enable the provisions of the Act to be applied effectively. As a result of this official guidance and encouragement nine of the Scottish local authorities within the next two years, invited the Board to give official sanction to their adoption of compulsory notification.

In England voluntary notification was begun in Brighton in January 1899, an example which was followed later in that year by Manchester and Sheffield. The latter city, under a local Act which came into operation in January 1904, changed over to compulsory notification, the first city in Britain to do so. These were, however, isolated instances and the first move from central authority was made in 1907 when the Local Government Board pronounced officially in favour of voluntary notification. A more positive step was taken in 1908 when the Board issued the Public Health (Tuberculosis) Regulations, making this compulsory from 1 January 1909 for patients under the care of Poor Law medical officers either at home or in Poor Law institutions.

But the battle for national recognition was not yet won and in this same year of 1908 the then Chief Medical Officer of the Local Government Board, who was also the reigning president of the Section of Epidemiology of the Royal Society of Medicine, had come to the conclusion

> that at present it would be inexpedient, unwise and of relatively little use to advise the general adoption of compulsory notification of phthisis. Public opinion is not ripe for this step, and such notification would remain to a large extent a dead letter.[7]

This proved to be the last stand against the inevitable and in May 1911 the Public Health (Tuberculosis in Hospitals) Regulations provided for the compulsory notification of all cases of pulmonary tuberculosis receiving treatment in public institutions. This was followed almost immediately by the Public Health (Tuberculosis) Regulations which extended compulsory notification, from 1 January 1912 to all cases of pulmonary tuberculosis while the cycle was finally completed when the notification of *all forms of tuberculosis* was made compulsory from 1 February 1913.

The culmination of the campaign for notification dovetailed very neatly into the events assoicated with one major milestone in British social history, the passage of the National Insurance Act (1911), which

7   *Ibid.* p. 349.

established the right of every insured person to free medical treatment. The constant propaganda from the voluntary organizations had alerted the political mind to the necessity for making provision within the Act for the special problems of tuberculosis and accordingly section sixteen required Insurance Committees

> to make arrangements with a view to providing treatment for insured persons suffering from tuberculosis (a) in sanatoria and other institutions, with persons or local authorities (other than poor law authorities) having the management of sanatoria or other institutions approved by the Local Government Board; (b) otherwise than in sanatoria or other institutions with persons and local authorities (other than poor law authorities) undertaking such treatment in a manner approved by the Local Government Board.

These intentions as set out in the Act were wholly admirable but one major obstacle lay in the way of their prompt translation into practice. In the years which had immediately preceded the passage of the Act a few of the more progressive local authorities had provided tuberculosis dispensaries but these were the exception. The majority of such dispensaries as existed had been established and maintained by voluntary effort, their number and the scope of their activities being governed by the finance available, while there was likewise a shortage of beds which were mainly in either privately owned or voluntary institutions. In both respects the total resources fell woefully short of what was obviously going to be required under the Act with its provisions for 'sanatorium benefit', and the Government appreciated the urgent need for a radical re-appraisal of the position. In order that a well thought-out plan, embracing all facets of the problem and applicable to the entire country, might be produced it was decided to set up, in February 1912, a Departmental Committee with the following terms of reference:

> To report at an early date upon the considerations of general policy in respect of the problems of tuberculosis in the United Kingdom, in its preventive, curative and other aspects which should guide the Government and local bodies in making or aiding provision for the treatment of tuberculosis in sanatoria or other institutions or otherwise.

The Committee was under the chairmanship of Waldorf Astor, MP (later Viscount Astor) and its members included Noel Bardswell, medical superintendent of the King Edward VII Sanatorium at Midhurst, Marcus Paterson, by then medical director of the King

Edward VII Welsh National Memorial Association, Arthur Latham (who, in addition to being physician at the Brompton Hospital, had had a large share in the planning of the Midhurst sanatorium), Arthur Newsholme and R. W. Philip.

The Committee got down to work immediately, for the 'sanatorium benefit' provided by the Act was to be available from 15 July and time, therefore, was of the essence. The time factor led to the decision to issue an interim report because, in the Committee's view,

> Preliminary arrangements will shortly have to be made, both centrally and locally, and the Committee deems it of great importance that any steps taken under that Act by any of the Authorities or bodies concerned should be in general harmony with the scheme which they desire to recommend. This report will, therefore, deal mainly with the essential features and broad lines of a comprehensive scheme with special reference to the practical steps which should be taken in the near future, for the provision of immediate treatment for the existing tuberculous population according to our present knowledge.[8]

The scheme recommended by the Committee placed the dispensary, modelled on that created by Philip in Edinburgh 25 years earlier, as the *first unit* in the national plan. It was to serve as a reception and diagnostic centre, as a clearing-house and as a centre for observation; it would also, in some instances, undertake curative treatment; contacts would be traced and examined through its agency; it would be responsible for 'after-care'; and would also act as a bureau for the education of the public in matters concerning tuberculosis. The *second unit* would consist of sanatoria and hospitals and here the Committee strongly recommended that the individual sanatorium should contain not less than 100 beds.

The Committee diverged from the Edinburgh plan, on two points, both important—the siting of the sanatoria and the staffing of the whole scheme. Philip believed that sanatoria should be located in the immediate vicinity of the large centres so that

> patients and the public should get rid of the prevalent but most erroneous belief that a cure can only be affected and health maintained under conditions which their ordinary residence and station in life will not permit them to enjoy.[9]

8 Departmental Committee on Tuberculosis (1912) *Interim Report.* p. 5. London: H.M.S.O.
9 Philip, R. W. (1) p. 52.

The Committee, while conceding that treatment could be carried out satisfactorily in sanatoria situated close to large centres of population, considered that such sites would prove costly and on grounds of expense, therefore, came down in favour of a more isolated position thus preparing the way for a host of administrative problems which were to grow in complexity over the years. Another conviction of Philip's was that the dispensary physician should have clinical charge of the associated institutions but the Committee elected to separate the functions of dispensary physician (tuberculosis officer) and sanatorium medical superintendent, a decision which gave rise to a narrowness of outlook and, at times, a conflict of interest on the part of both. The unfortunate dichotomy resulting from this ill-judged decision was not rectified until 1948.

One important recommendation in the interim report embodied the Committee's unanimous view that it was vital for the success of any scheme which might be adopted that it should apply to the whole community and should not be restricted, as envisaged in the Act, to insured persons and their dependents only. When they came to publish their Final Report in 1913 they were able to record with satisfaction that the Government had accepted this recommendation and had decided to place at the disposal of Local Government Boards an annual sum which would represent approximately half the cost of treating non-insured persons as well as the dependants of the insured.

The Final Report covered such diverse aspects of prevention as the protection of the milk supply and the special problem of tuberculosis in children. It also stressed, in its conclusion, the desirability and importance of allocating a proportion of the available resources to the financing of research projects.

The Committee gave its approval to a variation in respect of Wales. The King Edward VII Welsh National Memorial Association which had been founded in 1910 for the specific purpose of conducting the campaign against tuberculosis and on which was represented every local authority and insurance committee within the Principality, was to be permitted to continue to run its own affairs in its own way.

The recommendations of the Astor Committee were the foundations upon which the British tuberculosis service was built and until the middle of July 1914, substantial progress had been made by local authorities in setting up their schemes. Sir James Kingston Fowler summarized the situation throughout England then, as indicated in the following table.[10]

Number of schemes initiated by local authorities.

	County Councils (50)		County Boroughs (76)	
	Schemes Submitted	*Schemes Approved*	*Schemes Submitted*	*Schemes Approved*
Fairly complete schemes	39	37	60	53
Partial schemes	1	1	4	2
Dispensaries only	5	6	6	6
Total	45	44	70	61

But these encouraging developments were brought to a standstill in August 1914 by the outbreak of World War I when, as the national resources were mobilized for war, new schemes were held back and the building of sanatoria postponed. This check, although only temporary, was none the less serious, for tuberculosis was not to be denied its customary role as the concomitant of war and the toll which it exacted from its victims, service and civilians alike, presented a challenge to the newly fledged tuberculosis service in the later stages of the war and throughout the immediate post-war years.

While the British scheme was gradually evolving a similar process was taking place in the United States where Robert Philip had his counterpart in the person of Hermann M. Biggs. The operation which Biggs was to initiate centred on New York where, in 1889, in conjunction with Mitchell Prudden and H. P. Loomis, he submitted, at the request of the then City Commissioner of Health, Dr Joseph D. Bryant, a brief report on the contagiousness of tuberculosis which S. A. Knopf later described as marking 'the most important epoch in the control of tuberculosis in New York City as well as in the United States, if not in the entire civilized world.'[11] This report, as summarized by Winslow, made the following points:

1st That tuberculosis is a distinctly preventable disease.
2nd That it is not directly inherited; and
3rd That it is acquired by the direct transmission of the tubercle bacillus

10 Fowler, J. Kingston (1923) *Problems in Tuberculosis.* p. 7 London: Frowde & Hodder & Stoughton.
11 Knopf, S. A. (1922) A history of the National Tuberculosis Association. *N.Y. Nat. Tuberc. Ass.* p. 6.

from the sick to the healthy, usually by means of the dried and pulverized sputum floating as dust in the air.

The measures, then, which are suggested for the prevention of the spread of tuberculosis are:

1st The security of the public against tubercular meat and milk, attained by a system of rigid official inspection of cattle.

2nd The dissemination among the people of the knowledge that every tuberculous person may be an actual source of danger to his associates, if the discharges from the lungs are not immediately destroyed or rendered harmless and

3rd The careful disinfection of rooms and hospital wards that are occupied or have been occupied by phthisical patients.[12]

Commissioner Bryant, anxious to secure the acquiescence of the medical profession in any advice or directive which he might feel impelled to issue, submitted the report to 24 of the leading physicians in the city. Of these only two replied both favouring action along the lines suggested; the others, either through sheer indifference or hostility, did not trouble to answer. Biggs and his colleagues were therefore considerably in advance of contemporary medical thought and it is to Commissioner Bryant's credit that he elected to support their view and (in July 1889) issued a circular, prepared by Biggs for distribution both to physicians and laymen, entitled *Contagious Consumption—Rules to be Observed for the Prevention of the Spread of Consumption*. Thus the first step in the educational campaign against tuberculosis in the United States was taken and, having gained this advantage, Biggs pressed steadily on. In 1893 his dogged persistence carried the day when the New York Health Department adopted the Biggs programme which later served as the model for similar projects throughout the United States and Canada. This programme provided for

(1) a systematic campaign of public education calling attention to the dangers of the spread of tuberculosis, the possibilities of treatment, and the precautions necessary for its prevention; (2) the compulsory reporting of tuberculosis by all institutions while voluntary reporting was requested from all physicians in private practice; (3) the appointment of special inspectors to visit the homes of patients thus reported to enforce sanitary regulations regarding sputum disposal and disinfection; (4) advising general hospitals of the need to provide special wards for

12 Wimslow, C. E. A. (1929) *The Life of Hermann M. Biggs*. p. 86 Philadelphia: Lea & Febiger.

the reception of cases of pulmonary tuberculosis; (5) the establishment of a special hospital exclusively for the treatment of tuberculosis; (6) the provision of adequate laboratory facilities for the purposes of diagnosis.[13]

Still not wholly satisfied, Biggs succeeded over the subsequent decade in securing further important measures of control: the compulsory notification (in 1897) of all forms of tuberculosis, a scheme of public health nursing and home supervision, the establishment in 1904 of the first of a chain of clinics for diagnosis and treatment, the organization of a voluntary tuberculosis association designed to supplement the activities of the health department in the field of education and propaganda and the provision of adequate relief for tuberculous patients and their families to enable them to carry out the recommendations of the health department.

In essentials this programme differed but little from Philip's scheme in Edinburgh but, as both developed into national campaigns in their respective countries, certain differences became apparent. The constitution of the United States places the responsibility for public health matters on the sovereign states with intervention by the Federal Government only when these matters have an interstate or national significance. Consequently the Federal Government has never participated in tuberculosis control programmes other than by the provision of treatment facilities for certain special groups, such as ex-servicemen, and by research projects sponsored by the United States Public Health Service.

This relative absence of federal participation was one cause of the prominence given throughout America to the role of the voluntary tuberculosis association. For an understanding of this role it has to be appreciated that at the beginning of the twentieth century there were few well-organized public health departments throughout the country and in many communities it was necessary to lay the foundations of a public health programme before any progress could be made in tuberculosis control. There was a clear need for some organization capable of arousing public opinion to the point where community action became imperative and for this purpose the voluntary tuberculosis association, composed of representative citizens and supported entirely by voluntary contributions, appeared ideal. Such an association 'independent of public officialdom and local bureaucracy, and independently financed, is free not only to initiate and demonstrate

13 Jacobs, P. P. (1932) The control of tuberculosis in the United States. *N.Y. Nat. Tuberc. Ass.* pp. 5–7.

new procedures, but also to criticise and condemn if necessary the acts of public officials.[14]

Organized on municipal, county or state lines, voluntary tuberculosis associations sprang up in large numbers and gave representation on their directing boards to all groups who had a definite interest in tuberculosis:

> they are primarily responsible for stimulating the public purse to provide for the participation of official agencies in the tuberculosis campaign. The official, governmental participation and leadership in tuberculosis work is not taken for granted. It is not too much to say that without the non-official associations, the tuberculosis movement in the United States would have been greatly retarded and that the efficiency of the official agencies, dependant to a large extent upon the ever-watchful co-operation of these extra-governmental agencies, would be considerably impaired.[15]

In 1904 the National Association for the Study and Prevention of Tuberculosis (later to be re-named the National Tuberculosis Association), was founded under the presidency of Edward L. Trudeau and with William Osler and Hermann M. Biggs as vice-presidents. The new Association took up with enthusiasm the task of public education and later added to its functions co-ordination of the activities of local tuberculosis associations, organization of annual meetings and conferences and sponsoring of research programmes.

On the continent of Europe the pattern of attack on tuberculosis closely resembled that seen in Britain and in the United States, with voluntary associations initially playing the major part until they were supplemented, although not usually replaced by, the resources of the State.

In France the League against Tuberculosis had been founded in 1892 by Armingaud of Bordeaux while the first dispensary, the Émile-Roux Model Dispensary, was opened at Lille in 1901 by Professor Albert Calmette. In 1903 the famous Œuvre de la Preservation de l'Enfance contre la Tuberculose was initiated by J. Grancher after whom it later came to be named. Run as a private charity but receiving a government grant the 'Œuvre Grancher' arranged the boarding-out of young children from infected homes with healthy peasant families and in 1921 earned from Armand Delille the comment

14 *Ibid.* p. 11.
15 *Ibid.* p. 12.

that 'the Grancher system is at the same time the most useful, the least expensive, and the most radical and successful method of fighting tuberculosis.'[16]

The German Central Committee for combating tuberculosis was established in 1895 and the first centre for the dissemination of information regarding prevention was opened at Halle in 1899. By 1903 such centres had multiplied and had joined forces with the organization Fursorgestellen to care for the consumptive at home, to arrange for the examination of contacts and to remove young children from heavily infected homes. In 1904 the initial step in the development of the dispensary system was taken under the direction of Professor Kayserling at the Charité Hospital in Berlin.

In the Netherlands the Association for the Assistance of Persons of Dutch Nationality suffering from Lung Disease had been founded in 1897 followed a year later by the Association for Establishing and Conducting Public Sanatoria for Sufferers from Pulmonary Troubles. In 1902 the first public sanatorium was opened at Hellendoorn and the first dispensary at Rotterdam in 1903.

The campaign in Denmark was notable for the high degree of collaboration between voluntary and public agencies. The National Association for the Fight against Tuberculosis had been formed in 1901 and by 1903 was in a position to open three sanatoria. The Society of Danish Tuberculosis Physicians was founded in 1905 and in 1903 the National Association established the first chest clinic in Copenhagen. Denmark took a special pride in the contribution to treatment which stemmed from the discovery by Niels Finsen in 1892 of the curative influence of light upon lupus and the Finsen Institute, established in Copenhagen in 1895, grew rapidly into a hospital of considerable size with special departments for the treatment of all forms of extra-pulmonary tuberculosis.[17] Another worthy Danish contributor to the fight for prevention was Bernhard Bang who, in 1889, published his comprehensive studies on the spread of bovine tuberculosis. This work led up to the passing of the Danish Bovine Tuberculosis Act of 1898 which provided for the tuberculin testing of herds and for the slaughter, against compensation paid by the State, of all animals suffering from tuberculosis of the udder.

16 Delille, Armand (1921) (Quoted by Meachen, G. N. (1936)) *A Short History of Tuberculosis.* p. 74. London: J. Bale, Sons & Danielsson.
17 *The Fight against Tuberculosis in Denmark* p. 14. (1950) Danish National Association for the Fight against Tuberculosis.

In Norway much good work was done by the Norwegian National Association for Preventing Tuberculosis and the Norwegian Women's Health Association. Notification was made compulsory in 1901 and a dispensary system similar to that in Britain was planned in conjunction with the building of a number of national sanatoria.

The gathering momentum, all over the world, of the attack upon tuberculosis gave rise to a suggestion that an international society for the study of the disease and of methods for its prevention should be formed. The idea, first aired at a congress in Paris in 1898, led in 1902 to the formation of the International Central Bureau for the Campaign against Tuberculosis. This organization set up offices in Berlin from which, under the emblem of the double-barred cross, it undertook the planning and direction of the subsequent congresses which now developed into a regular feature of the international scene. In 1914 the International Central Bureau became another war casualty but it was destined to rise again in 1920 and, with permanent headquarters at Geneva and under its new name of the International Union against Tuberculosis, to play a prominent part in the stirring events which were to unfold in the middle decades of the century.

Chapter Twelve
Interlude—1914 to 1919

The impact of World War I on the emergent British tuberculosis service was immediate and disastrous. Many local authorities, anxious to implement the recommendations of the Astor Report as soon as possible, had prepared appropriate schemes: plans for new sanatoria had been considered and approved, suitable sites had been secured and only the final official blessing of the Local Government Board was required to enable the work to go ahead. At this point the Government decided that, because of the war, the building of sanatoria should cease and that all work on the various local authority schemes should be deferred. In addition a proportion of the existing hospitals and sanatoria was requisitioned by the War Office, thus imposing a further severe handicap on the service at the very moment when it was about to encounter the first major crisis of its brief career.

The plan which had been formulated for the ultimate provision of a tuberculosis-free milk supply also became an early casualty. The Tuberculosis Order of May 1913 had required the notification of cattle suffering from disease of the udder or from general tuberculosis with emaciation; it had laid down regulations governing the slaughter of affected animals and the payment of compensation and had thus marked the first real attempt in Britain to deal with the question of bovine tuberculosis. A further order followed in 1914 extending notification to all cattle with a chronic cough or with clinical signs of tuberculosis but this order was withdrawn on 6 August and, although under the Milk and Dairies (Consolidation) Act 1915, the sale of tuberculous milk was prohibited nothing further was done in this important matter until 1922.

For a time the antituberculosis campaign appeared to have ground to a halt but the temporary stagnation of these early war years provided the opportunity for some stock-taking and for a review of what had so far been accomplished. The Government and the public had put their faith in the sanatorium but it was becoming clear that there were aspects of the problem which could not be solved by sanatorium treatment alone if the criterion of success was to be the restoration of the patient's working capacity to the point where he could again support himself and his family. It required no great discernment to see that what was being achieved fell far short of this target. Any lingering sense of euphoria which might have pervaded the public mood was dissipated by the figures quoted by Varrier-Jones who had noted, from studies conducted on ex-sanatorium patients, that from 27 to 64 per cent died within five years of discharge, the main mortality occurring in the first two years. He declared also that in 75 per cent of the patients sent to sanatoria complete cure was out of the question, that the best to be expected was arrest of the disease and that, even then, this arrest was far from being permanent in over 50 per cent of cases.[1]

It was clear from such evidence that the patient recently discharged from a sanatorium was seldom if ever in a position to compete in the open market with his healthy fellow men and that, although a proportion of ex-patients might in time become fit enough to return to normal industry, the vast majority would require some special provision. Philip had anticipated the problem years previously and, admittedly greatly influenced by his obsession with the curative properties of fresh air, had added the farm colony to his co-ordinated scheme, describing it 'as a kind of postgraduate school suited to the requirements of a certain number of individuals who need more prolonged surveillance and direction than is convenient at the hospital'.[2] It did not seem that the farm colony could be of any significant assistance in the situation shown to exist by the figures of Varrier-Jones. A few patients sufficiently robust physically for the rigours of farm labour and the relative isolation of country life might benefit by a period of 'toughening up' in such a colony as a preliminary to a return to normal industry: for others schemes of vocational training for alternative occupations, conducted either within the curtilage of the sanatorium or in separate, designated centres, were advocated. There still remained a proportion for whom permanent sheltered employment appeared to be the only solution, either in

1 Varrier-Jones, P. C. (1943) *Papers of a Pioneer*. p. 15. London: Hutchinson.
2 Philip, R. W. (1937) *Collected Papers on Tuberculosis*. p. 141. London: Oxford University Press.

model workshops built for the purpose or—the ultimate in re-habilitation—within a village settlement.

The village settlement was a peculiarly British institution: it attracted much favourable comment by reason of two of its main aspects: the settlement of *both* the patient and his family in one village community and the provision of a variety of suitably light industries. The case for such settlements was well summed up by the man with whom the idea originated.

> If a man knew in the event of his being found to be tuberculous, that he would receive immediate treatment, that his family would be supported while he was receiving treatment, and that if he proved to be suffering from extensive and permanent damage he would be able to live and work permanently in a village settlement with his family, the whole tuberculosis problem would be revolutionized. Those who thought they had tuberculosis would present themselves for treatment at a very early stage and then our sanatoria would be able to report a far greater measure of success than is possible at the present time.[3]

The prototype of the village settlement, Papworth in Cambridge-shire, started in 1916 in the smallest possible way, its nucleus being an old country house, two acres of grounds and a few wooden shelters.[4] The brain-child of Dr (later Sir) Pendrill Varrier-Jones, Papworth Village Settlement was destined to grow into a large organization, to achieve considerable renown and to attract much publicity, due largely to the personality, administrative ability and remarkable talent for fund-raising of its founder. It is, nevertheless, debatable whether the results attained by Papworth could ever be said to have justified fully the expectations of its sponsors and the high hopes with which the scheme had been launched and it is probably significant that only one other similar project, at Preston Hall in Kent, was ever attempted.

In New York a serious effort to get to grips with the problem of resettlement was made in 1915 with the founding of the Altro Workshops. This organization provided work at garment making, in hygienic surroundings and under medical control, for patients with quiescent lesions of whom four out of five had had, at some time before entering employment, moderately advanced or far advanced disease. The hours of work were graduated in accordance with the

3 Varrier-Jones, P. C. (1931) The economics of after-care in tuberculosis. *Br. J. Tuberc.* 24, 175.
4 Varrier-Jones, P. C. (1) p. 45.

medical needs of each individual, being gradually increased until the limit of a seven-hour working day had been reached. The aim was the rehabilitation of the quiescent case rather than the provision of sheltered employment for the permanently disabled and a survey of the late results carried out in 1944 was considered to be excellent, 97.8 per cent of the 'graduates' being alive five years after discharge from the workshops.[5]

The whole question of the resettlement of the ex-sanatorium patient was generally regarded as posing particularly difficult problems, and in Britain it was to arise in an acute form at the end of the war and to be the subject of a report by a special inter-departmental committee set up by the Government.

The turmoil and turbulence of war was not calculated to create an environment conducive to serious scientific thought and study but in spite of the distractions around him K. E. Ranke in 1917 published his work on the evolution and pathogenesis of tuberculosis,[6] a subject which at that stage was still not clearly understood. As far back as 1876 Joseph Marie-Jules Parrot had announced at the Société de Biologie at Paris his 'law of similar adenopathies' according to which there was in the child no affection of the lungs which would not also be present in the adjoining lymph glands and likewise no change in the tracheobronchial lymph glands unaccompanied by a similar process within the lung.[7] Applying this law to tuberculosis Parrot had succeeded in demonstrating the primary lung focus in 145 cases of childhood tuberculosis examined postmortem at his children's hospital.

G. Küss returned to the subject in 1896 describing what later came to be termed the primary complex as 'a special form of tuberculosis in childhood which clinically cannot be diagnosed but can be detected at autopsy by minute examination'. He recognized this as the first stage of infection and noted its tendency to heal: he noted also that it could spread further and, sooner or later, end in a clinically recognizable form of tuberculosis

> by which the lungs can be affected by a retrograde movement through the lymphogenous, haematogenous and aspiratory channels and especially

5   Clarke, B. R. (1952) *Causes and Prevention of Tuberculosis*. p. 276. Edinburgh: E. & S. Livingstone.
6   Ranke, K. E. (1917) Primäres, Sekundäres und Tertiäres Stadium der Menschlichen Tuberkulose. *Berl. klin.-ther. Wschr. 54*, 397.
7   Parrot, J. M. J. (1876) (quoted by Ghon, A. (1916)) *The Primary Lung Focus of Tuberculosis in Children*. p. ix. (English trans. by D. B. King) London: Churchill.

in the apices of the lungs or the channels by which the tuberculous process in other cases localises itself secondarily in any other organ.[8]

Küss's work made little contemporary impact but in 1912 attention was drawn to it and due acknowledgement rendered by the Prague pathologist, Anton Ghon, who published his book on *The Primary Lung Focus of Tuberculosis in Children* in which he confirmed all the findings of Küss. Ghon's pathological studies, painstaking though they were, led to nothing new, other than the attachment of his own name to the pulmonary component of the primary complex (Ghon focus).

Thus far the exact relationship between the primary complex and the later manifestations of tuberculosis had remained obscure and it was an attempt to clarify this obscurity which led to Ranke's publication in 1917. He propounded a theory in which he postulated primary, secondary and tertiary stages in the development of tuberculosis and in which he linked each stage not only with the specific type of the organic lesion but also with the state of hypersensitivity and resistance of the infected individual. He agreed that the primary complex of Parrot, Küss and Ghon represented the starting point of the disease process, an opinion which met with general acceptance. His views on the development of the second stage encountered opposition since he maintained that every primary infection was succeeded by a secondary phase, characterized by marked tissue hypersensitivity, in which there was a diffuse dissemination of bacilli via the blood stream which distributed them widely throughout the body. This proposition provided a reasonable and acceptable explanation of the early post-primary phenomena of acute miliary tuberculosis and tuberculous meningitis. Many found it difficult to believe, as Ranke insisted that dissemination took place in every case although in the vast majority it was of mild degree and clinically abortive. The tertiary stage, that of increased resistance and reduced sensitivity, produced the pathological picture of isolated tuberculosis of a single organ or organ system, the form of disease with which both the public and the medical profession were most familiar. The development of this stage was ascribed to flare-up and progression of either the original primary focus or of one of the latent disseminated foci from a clinically abortive second stage or, alternatively, to the intervention of a fresh infection from without. Thus began an argument concerning the

8   Küss, G. (1898) *Ibid* p. xi.

respective frequency of 'endogenous exacerbation' and of 'exogenous superinfection' as the source of the tertiary lesion in tuberculosis, a debate which continued right up until the discovery of effective chemotherapy. Then the protagonists of the rival theories, accepting that the march of events had made the issue one of academic relevance only, decided to call it a day and, accepting that both possibilities could and did occur, refrained from any further attempts to apportion frequency or allocate priority.

Ranke's classification was heavily attacked as providing too facile an explanation without sufficient proof and as being subject to numerous exceptions and exclusions. Rich dismissed it in a few paragraphs[9] but Jaffe, commenting on an earlier pronouncement by Rich, held that the latter did 'not do full justice to this fundamental contribution'[10] while it is notable that such a great authority as Walter Pagel was to find Ranke's view acceptable.[11] Despite its critics Ranke's classification must be considered an historical landmark in the pathogenesis of tuberculosis and his views were ultimately to gain a much greater degree of acceptance than rejection.

By 1918 the clinical and administrative problems associated with tuberculosis were a matter for acute concern to the nations of Europe, where the tide of war was producing an abundant flotsam in the form of a steadily rising incidence of the disease. The figures make sombre reading: between 1913 and 1918 tuberculosis mortality rose by 17 per cent in England, 34 per cent in Italy, 44 per cent in Holland, 62 per cent in Germany and 30 per cent (until 1917) in Denmark.[12] There is ample evidence, accepted by virtually all authorities, that the main factor in the production of this increased mortality was malnutrition— a view supported by the figures from Denmark which, as a non-belligerent, escaped other contributory factors which were operating among the warring nations. Denmark existed mainly on the revenue derived from the export of meat and dairy products and, during the first years of the war, the demand for these by the belligerent powers was so great that, within Denmark, prices rose to unprecedented heights: unfortunately wages failed to keep pace with the rising prices

9   Rich, A. R. (1944) *The Pathogenesis of Tuberculosis*. pp. 750–2. Springfield, Ill.: Charles C. Thomas.
10   Jaffé, R. H. (1939) The pathology of pulmonary tuberculosis. In *Clinical Tuberculosis* (ed. B. Goldberg) Philadelphia: F. A. Davies.
11   Pagel, W., Simmonds, F. A. H., MacDonald N. & Nassau E. (1964) *Pulmonary Tuberculosis*. London: Oxford University Press.
12   Clarke, B. R. (5) p. 116.

and consequently the working class population had to endure an increasing food shortage. Parallel with this food shortage the tuberculosis mortality rose from 138 per 100 000 in 1914 to 176 per 100 000 in 1917, at which point the effects of the British blockade and of Germany's unrestricted submarine warfare combined to curtail severely Denmark's capacity to export and to import. The country was forced to live on its own produce, a shortage of feeding stuffs led to large-scale slaughtering of cattle and pigs and, as price control was introduced, the consumption of protein *per capita* rose to an acceptable level. This improved nutrition was immediately reflected in the tuberculosis figures, the mortality in 1918 reverting to 138 per 100 000 —as it had been in 1914.[13]

While the mortality figures in Britain were lower than those on the Continent, due to the ability of British seapower to ensure a reasonably adequate, even if far from lavish, food supply they were still sufficiently high to give rise to much anxiety, particularly in view of the restricted facilities available for treatment. Special concern was felt for tuberculous ex-servicemen who, by 1919, numbered some 35 000. Although these men had been given priority over the civilian population in respect of admission for residential treatment, the position remained unsatisfactory. Alarmed by the extent of the problem and goaded by the pressure of public opinion, the Government demonstrated its intention of grappling with the situation by the appointment of an Inter-Departmental Committee on Tuberculosis (Sanatoria for Soldiers)

to consider and report upon the immediate practical steps which should be taken for the provision of residential treatment for discharged soldiers and sailors suffering from tuberculosis and for their re-introduction into employment, especially on the land.

This Committee, like that of 1912, was under the chairmanship of Waldorf Astor but, owing to the pressure of Parliamentary business, he found it impossible to attend the meetings regularly and the report of the Committee was therefore signed by the Deputy Chairman, Sir Montague Barlow. His Committee's investigations revealed that of the 35 000 ex-servicemen suffering from tuberculosis, 22 000 had received or were currently receiving residential treatment 'which has often been for far too short a period'. The existing accommodation in the United Kingdom for adult males amounted to between 10 000

13 Rich, A. R. (9) p. 615.

and 11 000 beds and the serious shortage indicated by these figures was, in the Committee's opinion, the result of Government policy in suspending the building of sanatoria on the outbreak of war coupled with the requisitioning by the War Office for purposes of its own of a number of local hospitals and sanatoria. The Committee had no difficulty in reaching a decision to recommend an immediate increase in residential accommodation emphasizing that the provision of such accommodation for both ex-servicemen and civilians should be treated as one problem although ex-service personnel were still to be accorded priority in the allocation of beds.[14]

When it passed on to consider the second part of its remit—that dealing with the re-introduction into employment of the ex-servicemen—the Committee was clearly in difficulties. Memoranda regarding six training colonies, either existing or projected, were submitted in evidence and some of this evidence was conflicting. One positive point which did emerge fairly clearly was 'that agricultural work, training for which has been unduly emphasized in the past, is not generally suitable for those who have suffered from tuberculosis'[15] and such a forthright statement by the Committee was welcomed. The general idea of training colonies received a qualified endorsement but warm approval was forthcoming for the provision of permanent village settlements on the Papworth system and it was recommended that consideration be given to the establishment of ten such settlements in various parts of the country, each capable of accommodating from 200 to 250 men and, where necessary, their families.

The final section of the report provided an indication of the quandary in which the Committee found themselves over the problem of the re-introduction of these patients into employment since it dealt with suggestions that provision be made for the settlement of tuberculous ex-servicemen in the Dominions 'in which the climatic conditions are such as to be likely to aid in the cure of the disease'. Enquiries made on behalf of the Committee as to the likelihood of finding such a happy solution to Britain's problem produced the information that the Dominions had been one jump ahead and had thoughtfully introduced legislation which placed a ban on immigrants suffering from tuberculosis.

The Barlow Report was not an epoch-making document and its

14 Report of Inter-Departmental Committee on Tuberculosis. (1919) *Sanatoria for Soldiers*. London: H.M.S.O.
15 *Ibid*. p. 11.

findings and recommendations lacked the clear-cut precision of the earlier Astor Report. This is not meant as a criticism of the Committee but it is merely an indication of the much greater complexity of the problem with which it had been asked to deal. Eleven years later this problem was still defying solution as the extract from the 1931 report of the Employment Committee of the Joint Tuberculosis Council on *Care and After-Care Schemes in Tuberculosis* shows

> It is becoming increasingly evident that so-called employment schemes, as at present administered, handicraft classes, vocational therapy centres, training colonies and village settlements, can only give permanent employment to an insignificant number of cases in comparison with the magnitude of the problem as a whole. There are probably at least 15 per cent of all cases at any time which are purely medical problems and for whom employment of any kind is out of the question. The most reliable information shows that 40 to 50 per cent of cases return to their previous employment or to some modified branch of it. There remains therefore a balance of some 35 per cent who are both medical and economic responsibilities on the nation. It is for this group that employment schemes in tuberculosis should cater but the reporters have held strongly to the view that such schemes should be regarded as a means to the end rather than the end itself. Their function is to continue the healing process in a diseased lung and *not* to maintain a healed lesion in a state of perpetual innocence in a special community.[16]

Even after 1931 the rehabilitation and re-settlement of the tuberculous patient continued to provide the thorniest problem in the whole field of tuberculosis therapy and it is no reflection on the workers in that field, the experts as well as the purely well-intentioned, to admit that it was never really solved until the advent of effective chemotherapy put an end to the need for it.

16 Joint Tuberculosis Council (1931) *Care and After-Care Schemes in Tuberculosis.* Preston Hall, Aylesford, Kent: After-Care Department.

Chapter Thirteen
Post-war Resurgence

After the hiatus caused by World War I the battle against tuberculosis was resumed with energy and determination but there was still a span of a quarter of a century to be bridged before the discovery of effective chemotherapy—the discovery which was to revolutionize the whole plan of attack.

During these intervening years various countries proceeded with the organization of their tuberculosis services which, although varying in detail to accord with national practice and administrative structure, followed a similar basic pattern. The provision of facilities for diagnosis and treatment, the promotion of a campaign of prevention by intensive search for contacts, the planning of after-care for the recovering patient and the improvement of housing and of working conditions were universally recognized as essential.

These years saw the heyday of the sanatorium and the expansion and elaboration of collapse therapy with the thoracic surgeon ultimately becoming a fully accredited member of the therapeutic team. Radiology at last became recognized as an indispensable adjunct to the dispensary and the sanatorium, while later the development of tomography added a new dimension to the exploration of living lung pathology. These were exciting years for those who worked in the specialty for they witnessed the gradual dispersal of the clouds of despair which had hitherto cast their shadow over the victims of of tuberculosis, a proportion of whom could now be rescued by judiciously timed and skilfully performed pneumothorax and thoracoplasty.

In Britain progress resumed its march with the passing by Parliament of the Public Health (Tuberculosis) Act 1921 which imposed upon the local authorities—county councils and county borough councils—a duty to provide schemes for the treatment and after-care of tuberculosis within their areas. The onus of creating a British tuberculosis service along the lines laid down in the Astor Report was thereby placed squarely on their shoulders and plans which had had to be put into cold storage on the outbreak of war were taken out, refurbished and their introduction begun. By 1923 implementation had reached the point where there were, throughout England and Wales, 442 tuberculosis dispensaries staffed by 349 tuberculosis officers,[1] figures which suggested a willingness on the part of the local authorities to meet their obligations. The extensive national organization which was thus built up appeared impressive and doubtless gave satisfaction to those with whom the idea had originated. There were, nevertheless, inherent defects in the plan which became increasingly obvious with time and which were such as to make it virtually impossible for the organization to cope adequately with the enormous demands made upon it.

The scheme was based on the assumption that tuberculosis stood alone as a special problem, a view which was understandable at the time; but unfortunately the structure of the plan provided for the virtual isolation of this one disease from the general body of medicine. This was not so comprehensible and was to place the whole service at an unnecessary and increasing disadvantage. The tuberculosis dispensaries were established, not within the grounds of general hospitals (which would have been both logical and helpful to their future development), but most commonly in converted houses, hastily adapted for their new role and inadequately equipped for its fulfilment. Where new buildings were authorized the tendency was to reduce costs by the erection of purely functional structures which gave no sense of pride to those who worked in them and provided little bodily comfort for the attending patients. The situation was aggravated further, and the severance from general medicine completed, by adherence to the recommendation of the Astor Committee that, on grounds of economy, sanatoria should be sited in the more remote areas where building land was cheap. This policy of isolating both units of the scheme from the broad stream of general medicine and surgery not only deprived the staff of the stimulus of medical and social contacts but also hampered the development of thoracic surgery, of pathology and of radiology, all of which were to increase both in importance and in complexity during the years ahead. Separation from general medicine also created difficulties in the recruitment of medical staff of the requisite calibre, for the able and the ambitious saw the tuberculosis service as a backwater where, after a life spent in dealing with a chronic and notoriously

1 Fowler, J. K. (1923) *Problems in Tuberculosis*. p. 8. London: Hodder & Stoughton.

unresponsive disease, the peak of attainment would be an appointment as a senior tuberculosis officer or as the medical superintendent of a sanatorium. This problem was overcome in part by the tendency of physicians whose own planned careers had been wrecked by tuberculosis to enter the service on their recovery, a mutually beneficial arrangement which brought into the field of tuberculosis work many notable personalities whose crusading enthusiasm and professional ability did something to rescue the service from the mediocrity which was an inevitable result of strict adherence to the Astor Committee's dictates.

The policy of isolation from general medicine had repercussions on medical education as well and, in 1923, Sir James Kingston Fowler was gravely concerned over the inadequate instruction which students received in the physical diagnosis of the disease.

> When a Tuberculosis Department under the charge of a competent physician is to be found at every General Hospital to which a Medical School is attached . . . and the students make use of it, there will be fewer errors in diagnosis and a great many more doctors who can tell you where they 'learnt their chests'.[2]

The Edinburgh medical school had already taken the important step of creating a chair of tuberculosis, an example which was followed a few years later by the Welsh National School of Medicine, with the foundation of the David Davies chair, but in general the English medical schools showed little interest and at undergraduate level tuberculosis remained a much neglected subject.

These were some of the clinical deficiencies of the scheme but it would be idle to pretend that, these apart, it represented a planners' triumph. The delegation of organization to the local authorities, which may have appeared administratively convenient at the planning stage, produced many anomalies and inconsistencies in practice. The responsible authorities varied greatly in size and in financial resources with the result that some of the smaller and poorer areas, where the need for an adequate tuberculosis service was greatest, were unable to provide sufficient facilities. This inability was to give rise to increasing unevenness in the quality of the service as the more frequent use of collapse therapy, coupled with the employment of more sophisticated radiological techniques, necessitated increases both in staff and in specialized equipment. In only a few instances was the obvious answer of amalgamation adopted: the majority, cut off from

2 *Ibid.* p. 26.

154

this common sense solution by local rivalry and a mistaken civic pride, continued as isolated and relatively ineffective units until the situation was rectified by the regionalization programme of the new National Health Service in 1948. By way of contrast some of the larger and more progressively minded authorities, outstanding examples of which were Middlesex and Lancashire, organized and maintained schemes of a superlative efficiency which were able to hold their own with any in the world, while the exemption of Wales from certain provisions of the Astor Report and the operations of the Welsh National Memorial Scheme provided a preview of some of the benefits which could accrue from regionalization.

The main voluntary hospitals, such as the Brompton and the London Chest Hospital, although outside the national scheme made a notable contribution to overall progress in terms of research and in the initiation of advances in treatment, notably in the field of thoracic surgery.

In the United States the foundation of the National Tuberculosis Association in 1904 and the choice of Washington as the venue for the Sixth International Congress on Tuberculosis had done much to arouse public interest and thereafter an impressive array of state and local programmes were built up between 1908 and 1920. In 1917 the Transactions of the National Tuberculosis Association recorded that

> Starting with a handful of members, mostly on the Atlantic coast, and with practically no local or state associations except in a few eastern states and cities, we are able to report that at least we have reached one of the goals for which we have striven, namely, an active state anti-tuberculosis association in every state of the Union and also in a number of our outlying insular possessions such as Porto Rico, the Phillipine Islands, the Canal Zone and Hawaii.[3]

The absence of any co-ordinated national plan for the control of tuberculosis, allied to the considerable diversity of population and resources to be found throughout the United States, resulted in each state, city or county creating the type of tuberculosis programme which it felt was best suited to its own needs and within the range of what it could afford. In some areas the municipal or county authorities took the initiative, in others the voluntary associations led the campaign with the backing of the official authority, and throughout the country very substantial progress was made. By 1931 there were in the United States 633 tuberculosis hospitals and sanatoria with a total

3   Transactions of the National Tuberculosis Association (1917) *N.Y. Nat. Tuberc. Ass.* p. 29.

bed capacity of 80 054 of which 78 per cent were in publicly supported institutions, while the number of voluntary antituberculosis associations had risen to 1471. Out-patient facilities had not increased at the same rate and by 1928 there were no more than 1000 dispensaries or permanently sited clinics but these were being supplemented by the extensive employment of travelling and occasional clinics which, during that year, had provided 2500 out-patient sessions.[4]

Throughout the Continent the campaign followed a pattern which was similar in many respects to the British plan. Notification was made compulsory in Bulgaria, Denmark, Spain, Estonia, the Irish Republic, Iceland, Italy, Lithuania, Norway, Poland and the U.S.S.R., but remained optional in France, while in Germany it was required in respect of sputum-positive patients only.[5] Most countries had organized a dispensary system, the number of dispensaries provided being dependent on a variety of circumstances among which density of population, transport facilities and the availability of trained personnel were of major importance. Information collected by McDougall showed that, before the outbreak of World War II, the allocation of dispensaries in proportion to population was as follows:[6]

The allocation of dispensaries in proportion to population.

Country	Thousands of population for every one dispensary
Germany	45
Austria	80
Great Britain	84
Bulgaria	880
France	64
Holland	57
Hungary	140
Norway	533
Poland	148
Sweden	27
Switzerland	363
Czechoslovakia	85.7

4 Jacobs, P. P. (1932) The control of tuberculosis in the United States. *N.Y. Nat. Tuberc. Ass.* pp. 20–2.
5 McDougall J. B. (1949) *Tuberculosis. A Global Study in Social Pathology.* p. 383 Edinburgh: E. & S. Livingstone.
6 *Ibid.* p. 390.

All the evidence both from the Old World and the New now indicated a widespread awareness of the threat to health, happiness and prosperity that tuberculosis presented. The creation of an administrative structure directed towards its control, and the consequent increase in dispensaries and sanatoria, stimulated anew the search for more effective methods of treatment and it was to this quest that physicians and surgeons devoted their energies during the 1920s and 30s—20 years of fascinating collaboration in which much ingenuity was displayed and a great deal accomplished.

Chapter Fourteen
The High Noon of Collapse Therapy and Resection Surgery

The immediate post-war years saw the beginning of the boom in collapse therapy that was to dominate the treatment of pulmonary tuberculosis for the next quarter of a century. At first collapse therapy and artificial pneumothorax were virtually synonymous terms and, although alternative methods later became available, pneumothorax, largely because of the deceptive simplicity of its technique, continued to lead the field despite, in the 1940s, an increasing barrage of criticism and misgivings. In 1921 Sir James Kingston Fowler is on record as having stated that he 'had lived to see two real advances in the treatment of pulmonary tuberculosis, one sanatorium treatment and the other artificial pneumothorax'. In 1959, in what must have been one of the very last clinical papers written on artificial pneumothorax, Gosta Birath, a distinguished Swedish physician, opened with a quotation from an unidentified source to the effect that 'the pneumothorax needle was the most dangerous weapon ever placed in the hands of a physician'.[1] At the times when these sharply contrasting statements were made each contained much truth and the explanation of the revolt against pneumothorax, which is implicit in the 1959 comment, must be sought in a study of the manner in which it was practised throughout the intervening years.

But in 1922 hopes were high and the British Medical Research Council deemed it opportune to ask for a special report 'for making judgement of the remedial value of artificial pneumothorax—that method of treating disease of a lung by giving it controllable periods of rest from respiratory movement', a report which Dr L. S. T. Burrell, physician to the Brompton Hospital, and Dr A. S. Macnalty, a medical officer of the Ministry of Health, were invited to prepare.

---

1 Birath, G. (1959) The place of pneumothorax in the present day management of pulmonary tuberculosis. *Dis. Chest. 35*, 1.

Their report, published on 21 June 1922,[2] provided an admirable summary of current thinking since, in order to obtain 'a concensus of opinion not only as to the value of the treatment but also as to its indications and contraindications' it embodied the answers to a questionnaire circulated to 16 physicians associated with well-known hospitals or sanatoria. The 16 were unanimous in describing artificial pneumothorax as a notable therapeutic achievement and they reported beneficial results in between 50 and 60 per cent of patients in whom it had been successfully induced. That was however, the single point on which unanimity was reached.

A question on indications for the treatment elicited a particularly broad spectrum of opinion. Two physicians saw the method solely as a palliative measure for the really advanced case while two others urged that it be employed in the early stages, one declaring that in his view no case was 'too early' for this treatment. The remainder adopted a middle of the road policy in reserving it for patients with unilateral disease who were not responding to sanatorium treatment. All recognized the problem presented by pleural adhesions and the extent to which these could interfere with an effective lung collapse but only one had attempted, or even considered, adhesion section.

There was considerable variation also in plans for dealing with the complications of the treatment such as pleural effusion but no definite opinions were expressed on the significance of the latter. Claud Lillingston, who was among the 16, had added an important proviso to his reply:

> The differences in the results achieved at different institutions are almost completely to be explained by the differences in the skill and conscientiousness of the physician in charge.

The validity of this point was to become increasingly obvious during the years that lay ahead.

While the report gave a considerable impetus to pneumothorax therapy it also provided a foretaste of the factors which were to bedevil the procedure throughout all the years of its employment and which were to make the accumulation of readily comparable statistics virtually impossible. Lack of uniformity in case selection, divergence of view on what constituted an effective collapse, variation in policy regarding adhesion section and in the degree of concern

2 Burrell, L. S. T. & Macnalty, A. S. (1922) Report on artificial pneumothorax. *Med. Res. Council Special Report Series.* London: HMSO.

with which common complications such as chronic pleural effusion and empyema were viewed, all combined to impede the accurate comparison of results from different units and hence the formulation of reliable conclusions about the merits of the treatment. The natural history of most new surgical discoveries (and pneumothorax, although it came to be practised almost wholly by physicians, must be regarded as essentially a surgical manoeuvre) follows a fairly constant pattern—an initial period of caution and doubt is succeeded by over-enthusiasm and excessive use until ultimately reason and experience prevail and the discovery is either discarded as a failure or retained to deal with specific situations within a framework of recognized and accepted indications and contraindications. Artificial pneumothorax had passed through the greater part of the first phase in the years immediately preceding the Medical Research Council's Report and thereafter discretion was gradually thrown to the winds, ushering in a period of increasing utilization, often with scant regard being paid to indications or to the formidable complications which followed its misuse.

Unfortunately, and for a variety of reasons, this intermediate phase proved to be remarkably protracted. Lured on by the relative technical simplicity of both induction and maintenance and impelled by the understandable desire to do something active in the treatment of a killing disease, physicians were reluctant to accept the existence of very definite contraindications to pneumothorax. Of even greater importance was the failure of many to learn and apply two basic rules which were essential to its effective and safe use; that closed intrapleural pneumonolysis formed an indispensable part of this method of collapse; and that inability to divide adhesions or the onset of pleural complications were danger signals which called for its immediate abandonment. For a time, of course, developments were hampered by a lack of facilities for adhesion section and for alternative forms of collapse therapy but, once the demand had been created, the facilities became available although it is doubtful whether the extent of their availability, in either Britain or in the United States, was ever really adequate for the problem.

On the mainland of Europe the new specialty of thoracic surgery had been making greater strides and the names of German, Swiss, and Scandinavian surgeons were becoming familiar in the world literature. By the early 1930s most countries could point to their own acknowledged experts in the operation of closed intrapleural pneumonolysis.

Jacobaeus and Gravesen dominated the Scandinavian scene and Unverricht the German, while in Davos Gustav Maurer, with his own particular combination of energy and enthusiasm, devised new instruments and developed fresh techniques. In the United States R. C. Matson at Portland, Oregon, Welles at Saranac Lake and Alexander at Ann Arbor, Michigan, were among the early leaders in the field. In Britain Morriston Davies was under no illusions about the problem of pleural adhesions or about the need for an aggressive attitude towards its solution. His own early efforts at pneumonolysis were restricted to the attempted division of band-like adhesions, carried out under fluoroscopic control, by means of a long double-edged tenotome passed through an intercostal space, but he was glad to abandon this somewhat hazardous undertaking when the Jacobaeus thoracoscope became available.[3] Unfortunately some other leading British exponents of pneumothorax treatment showed less enlightenment and Clive Rivière of the London Chest Hospital undoubtedly retarded progress when, even in 1927, he regarded favourably a policy of 'stretching' adhesions by means of frequent refills with gradually increasing intrapleural pressures, a plan which he considered would be so successful that the Jacobaeus operation would only rarely be indicated.[4] A different view prevailed at the Brompton Hospital where, in 1924, Tudor Edwards published the first paper from a British hospital on the use of thoracoscopy in diseases of the chest.[5] Later, at the London Chest Hospital, a physician, Frederick George Chandler, led the way after he had designed a combined thoracoscope and cautery in contrast to the separate instruments favoured by Jacobaeus.[6] Throughout his career Chandler remained faithful to his combined instrument but, like the somewhat similar thoracoscope introduced by L. R. Davidson in the United States,[7] it found little favour with others.

By the late 1930s there had been a significant increase in the number of centres equipped to undertake closed intrapleural pneumonolysis, but it would be idle to pretend that everything was well and un-

3 Davies, H. M. (1924) Surgery in the treatment of pulmonary tuberculosis. *Br. med. J.* 2, 1145.
4 Rivière, C. (1927) *Pneumothorax and Surgical Treatment of Pulmonary Tuberculosis.* p. 78. London: Oxford University Press.
5 Edwards, A. T. (1924) Thoracoscopy in surgery of the chest. *Br. J. Surg. 12,* 69.
6 Chandler, F. G. (1930) A new thoracoscope. *Lancet, 1,* 232.
7 Davidson, L. R. (1929) A simplified operating thoracoscope. *Amer. Rev. Tuberc. 19,* 306.

profitable to speculate on all the reasons for the atmosphere of vague unease surrounding the whole question of pneumothorax therapy which was becoming apparent from 1940 onwards. It is, nevertheless, reasonable to conclude that one of the causes of this concern stemmed from failure to exploit fully the potentialities of adhesion section. That it was not being fully utilized appeared clear from the researches of Drolet who found in 1941 that in the United States pneumonolysis had been employed in only 2571 out of 17 221 pneumothorax patients in 101 representative sanatoria.[8] This represented 15 per cent of patients, a figure which appeared inadequate when considered in relation to the proportion in whom adhesions were known to be preventing an effective collapse, a proportion which varied from 45 to 82 per cent in a series of reports published between 1939 and 1941.[9, 10, 11] Cullen and Hoffman added emphasis to that view in 1942 with their uncompromising statement:

> Ample opportunity to compare pneumothorax with and without facilities for pneumonolysis has shown that pneumothorax, unaided by supplementary procedures, with pneumonolysis as the procedure of choice, is an inadequate measure in the treatment of pulmonary tuberculosis. Here we have an example when the expression 'halfway measures have no place' takes on meaning: pneumothorax without pneumonolysis, when indicated, is decidedly a half-way measure.[12]

The widespread employment of pneumothroax had resulted in a voluminous literature, yet in 1941 Robert Bloch, W. B. Tucker and W. E. Adams, after studying 2100 papers published during the decade 1929–39, noted that only 4.7 per cent of these were concerned with the *results* of the treatment. Pursuing the matter still further they reviewed the literature from 18 different countries covering *in toto* the period from 1918 to 1939 and discovered 99 papers featuring results. After formulating what they considered to be adequate and acceptable standards for the reporting of such results in order to 'obtain more reliable figures on the actual curative value of the treatment' they grouped the 99 papers according to their assessment of the standards

8 Drolet, G. J. (1943) Collapse therapy. *Amer. Rev. Tuberc. 47*, 184.
9 Jones, H. A. (1939) Closed intrapleural pneumonolysis. *Amer. Rev. Tuberc. 40*, 722.
10 Mattill, P. M. & Jennings, F. L. (1940) Accidents and complications of artificial pneumothorax. *Amer. Rev. Tuberc. 41*, 38.
11 Diamond, S. & Ivey, H. (1941) Pneumothorax in patients over forty. *Amer. Rev. Tuberc. 43*, 475.
12 Cullen, V. F. & Hoffman, R. (1942) Tuberculosis in the negro. *Amer. Rev. Tuberc. 45*, 53.

which had been adopted by the individual authors. Only in 34 per cent of these papers were the standards regarded as acceptable, the remainder being classified as either 'partially adequate', 'inadequate' or as being based on 'incomplete information'.[13] This work of Bloch and his colleagues is quoted merely to illustrate the difficulties which beset the path of the seeker after the truth about pneumothorax, difficulties which were to persist until the very end when the treatment was finally discarded with the advent of effective chemotherapy.

In 1944 a determined attempt was made by T. N. Rafferty to rescue artificial pneumothorax from the morass of doubt and contradiction in which it was floundering. His monograph on the subject contained a masterly exposition of all the rules, backed by cogent and irrefutable arguments, for the correct use of pneumothorax and he even carried his crusade to the point of declaring that, in certain circumstances, primary thoracoplasty was to be preferred as the first line of attack.[14] Such a policy was indeed a break with tradition, tradition which had the backing of the great authority of John Alexander, for hitherto it had been virtually axiomatic that pneumothorax should always be attempted before resorting to thoracoplasty even though such a course might well add the burden of pleural complications to an already serious situation. Had Rafferty's rules been accepted and followed meticulously the doubts which overshadowed pneumothorax therapy would almost certainly have been resolved. Unfortunately his work was read mainly by the converted rather than by that body of physicians, of highly varying degrees of competence, who believed that the only necessary qualification for the practice of pneumothorax was the ability to introduce air into the chest.

Evidence that the limitations of pneumothorax had been recognized at a fairly early stage is furnished by the story of the efforts which were directed towards devising other procedures which would either replace or supplement it. Some of these were either revivals or modifications of earlier ideas while one or two were new.

Extrapleural Pneumothorax. This operation consisted of the separation of the lung and pleurae from the thoracic wall, the extrapleural space thus created being maintained by the insertion of a filling substance. Tuffier, with whom the idea had originated in 1891,

13 Bloch, R. G., Tucker, W. B. & Adams, W. E. (1941) Standards and criteria in artificial pneumothorax therapy. *J. thorac. Surg., 10*, 310.
14 Rafferty, T. N. (1944) *Artificial Pneumothorax in Pulmonary Tuberculosis*. London: W. Heinemann.

was by 1910 employing fat as his filling material,[15] while in 1913 Baer introduced a 'plombe' of solid paraffin wax which, after warming, could be moulded into the required shape.[16] 'Apicolysis with plombage' for a time enjoyed a modest vogue in Continental clinics but it was never popular in Britain where there was resistance to the idea of introducing a foreign body such as paraffin into the tissues while British surgeons never learnt to accept with equanimity the disquieting frequency with which late extrusion of the paraffin through the scar occurred followed by a troublesome infection of the extrapleural space. In 1936, when plombage had lost much of its attraction, Graf of Dresden and Schmidt of Heidelberg proposed and carried out air refills of the extrapleural space,[17] extrapleural pneumothorax in its truest sense, and for a brief period this idea evoked an enthusiastic response both in Europe and in the United States. Theoretically it had much to commend it but there were practical disadvantages. The incidence of infection of the extrapleural air space—either tuberculous or pyogenic—was high; significant postoperative extrapleural haemorrhage was not unknown; and there was a pronounced tendency for the space to shrink and obliterate necessitating frequent refills with high pressures or the substitution of oil for air which was both messy and unsatisfactory. The disadvantages ultimately dampened the enthusiasm of even the most ardent advocates of extrapleural pneumothorax and by 1945 it had largely vanished from the therapeutic scene.

The final episode in the saga of the extrapleural space saw a reversion to plombage with the employment of either spheres or sponges made from inert plastic material. This procedure was rapidly displaced by a combination of chemotherapy and resection but not before a study by Trent and his colleagues at Duke Hospital in North Carolina had concluded that the results obtained did not justify its continuance.[18]

Oleothorax. Defined by Packard, Hayes and Blanchet as 'a form of

15 Tuffier, T. (1923) Collapstherapie par décollement pleuro-parietal pour tuberculose limitée au sommet du poumon, greffe d'un fragment de tissue adipeux dans l'espace décollé. *Bull. Soc. Chir. Paris, 49,* 1249.

16 Baer, G. (1913) Ueber extrapleurale Plombierung bei Lungentuberkulose. *Munch. med. Wschr., 60,* 1587.

17 Reid, H. (1952) Extrapleural pneumolysis. In *Modern Practice in Tuberculosis.* 87. Vol. 2, London: Butterworth.

18 Trent, J. C., Moody, J. D. & Hiatt, J. S. (1949) An evaluation of extrapleural pneumolysis with lucite plombage. *J. thorac. Surg., 18,* 173.

pulmonary collapse therapy produced by the introduction of oil into the pleural cavity'[19] the idea of oleothorax as a serious contribution to treatment was first put forward by A. Bernou.[20] It had a chequered career and amongst the indications for its use were (1) to prevent the premature re-expansion of a collapsed lung by the substitution of oil for air refills (2) to exert more constant compression on a thick walled cavity than that which was possible by air alone and (3) to treat a tuberculous empyema which was complicating an artificial pneumothorax. Its efficacy in the first situation was unpredictable while in the second and the third the attendant risks were high and the possible advantages extremely dubious. Other than by providing a good illustration of the straits to which physicians could be reduced in dealing with an ineffective or complicated pneumothorax it is of little interest and never enjoyed any large measure of general favour.

Phrenic Paralysis. Diaphragmatic paralysis was to play a much more prominent role in the story of collapse therapy than either plombage or oleothorax. Suggested by Stuertz in 1911 as a possible means of producing pulmonary relaxation in predominantly lower lobe lesions where artificial pneumothorax had failed, it was originally considered to involve mere division of the main phrenic nerve trunk or, at the most, resection of a short portion of the nerve. Later observations by Felix,[21] indicating that in a proportion of cases diaphragmatic function remained unimpaired despite section of the nerve, led to the discovery of accessory branches within the thorax, and to a re-appraisal of technique. Thereafter simple division of the main nerve was replaced either by 'radical' phrenicotomy when the accessory branches were also divided or by evulsion in which, after division, the distal portion of the main trunk was, by the exercise of steady traction, plucked from its insertion into the diaphragm and drawn out of the thorax bringing with it the accessory fibres. Both operations produced permanent paralysis of the diaphragm, a result which was later seen to have disadvantages and the, by then, popular phrenic evulsion was largely replaced by the phrenic 'crush' in which maceration of the nerve with artery forceps induced a temporary paralysis of approximately six months duration.

19 Packard, E. N., Hayes, J. N. & Blanchet, S. F. (1940) *Artificial Pneumothorax*. p. 237. London: H. Kimpton.
20 Bernou, A. (1922) L'oleothorax thérapeutique. *Bull. Acad. Méd., 87*, 457.
21 Felix, W. (1922) Anatomische, experimentelle und klinische Untersuchungen über den Phrenikus und über die Zwerchfellinnervation. *Dt. Z. chir., 171*, 283.

The operation of phrenic paralysis enjoyed much popularity throughout the whole era of collapse therapy. Its virtues were, perhaps, also its chief disadvantages. It was relatively simple to perform and, so long as a knowledge of the anatomy of the neck was combined with a modicum of ordinary surgical care, was remarkably free from complications. It appealed to the patient in that it represented positive action which also carried the cachet of a surgical operation and it had no long-term inconveniences such as the refills of a pneumothorax. With all this in its favour it was perhaps inevitable that the limited objective of lower lobe lesions for which it had been introduced was soon cast aside and that during the early 1930s, the indications for the operation were extended beyond all reason until they included virtually every type of lesion which pulmonary tuberculosis might produce.

In 1931 Edward J. O'Brien of Detroit reported a series of 500 cases (with apologies for omitting a further 200 where the operation had been too recent to permit of statistical analysis) and claimed beneficial results in 82 per cent of those which had presented with cavitation. Reports such as this led to an acute outbreak of phrenic operations and this widespread use naturally gave rise to much divergence of opinion as to its value. Those surgeons who had employed it in long-standing and advanced disease condemned it as ineffective while others, who had restricted its use to early cases, were enthusiastic about the benefits and overlooked the possibility that a proportion would have recovered satisfactorily without it. Between these two extremes there were, fortunately, surgeons whose clinical judgment and appreciation of the limitations of such a relatively minor procedure led them to employ it with discrimination, most frequently as part of a planned programme of combined collapse therapy rather than as definitive treatment in its own right, and it was in such a supplementary role that it came eventually to find its greatest usefulness.[22]

Pneumoperitoneum. The idea of using an artificial pneumoperitoneum as a means of providing relaxation for a diseased lung appears to have occurred first to Vadja when, in 1933, he introduced 1200 cc and 700 cc of air respectively into the peritoneal cavities of two patients with pulmonary tuberculosis[23] and noted the subsequent

22 Thorburn, G. & Riggins, H. M. (1941) Temporary phrenic paralysis in selected cases of partially effective pneumothorax. *Trans. natn. Tuberc. Ass. N.Y. 37*, 146.
23 Vadja, L. (1933) Ob das Pneumoperitoneum in die Kollapstherapie bei beiderseitigen Lungentuberkulose angewandt werden kann? *Z. Tuberk., 67* 371.

elevation of the diaphragms with the accompanying decrease in the amplitude of their excursions. In neither instance did he attempt to maintain the pneumoperitoneum but he did suggest that it might have therapeutic possibilities when adhesions prevented pneumothorax or, as a short-term measure, for the control of haemoptysis. The same proposal was made, also in 1933, by Andrew L. Banyai of Milwaukee after an incident in which, on attempting to establish a pneumothorax, he accidentally induced a pneumoperitoneum.[24] In 1936 Fremmel suggested that phrenic paralysis and pneumoperitoneum might profitably be combined,[25] a possibility which was also envisaged at about the same time by Joannides and Schlack.[26] Over the next few years pneumoperitoneum, usually but not exclusively in association with phrenic paralysis, was launched throughout the world—at a propitious moment since it coincided with the onset of the gradual fall from favour of pneumothorax. Pneumoperitoneum was admittedly less effective than the latter but it was also singularly free from the complications and misfortunes to which the pneumothorax patient was so prone and, used in conjunction with phrenic paralysis, it formed a combination which earned for itself a definite place in any planned programme of collapse therapy. Although occasionally employed as the sole measure of treatment this combination was more often the prelude to major surgery and with its aid many a poor operative risk was converted into one which was surgically acceptable.

Cavity Drainage. Although drainage of tuberculous cavities carries no entitlement to the term 'collapse therapy', it is included in this Chapter for reasons both of convenience and chronology. Originally proposed by de Cérenville in 1885 it appeared to lack surgical appeal and thereafter aroused only occasional and always quite transient interest until 1937 when Leo Eloesser attempted closed drainage of such cavities by the introduction of a tube through the chest wall and the application of suction.[27] He did not regard the results as satisfactory and, after a short trial, abandoned the idea.

24 Banyai, A. L. (1933) Direct and indirect pneumoperitoneum incidental to artificial pneumothorax. *Am. J. med. Sci. 186*, 513.
25 Fremmel, F. (1937) Phrenicectomy reinforced by pneumoperitoneum. *Am. Rev. Tuberc. 36*, 488.
26 Joannides, M. & Schlack, O. C. (1936) Use of phrenic neurectomy combined with artificial pneumoperitoneum for collapse of adherent tuberculous lung. *J. thorac. Surg., 6*, 218.
27 Eloesser, L. (1937) Quoted by Maxwell, R. J. C. & Kohnstamn, M. L. (1943) The transpleural drainage of tuberculous cavities. *Br. J. Tuberc. 37*, 24.

It was taken up by Monaldi, working at the Carlo Forlanini Institute in Rome, who evolved a theory, elaborated a technique and, for a time, popularized the method, particularly on the Continent.[28] He based his treatment on the conception that, while tissue destruction was initially responsible for the formation of a lung cavity, its further growth and persistence were due less to biological than to mechanical factors, the chief of these being its inflation, by air trapped under tension within it, distal to an inflamed and partially obstructed draining bronchus. Monaldi believed that the creation of a negative intracavitary pressure would overcome this tension leading to shrinkage of the cavity and ultimately to its closure, when the space which it had formerly occupied would be filled by the re-aeration of the compressed and atelectatic tissue which had formed the cavity wall, together with compensatory emphysema of the surrounding area of lung. He was careful to stress that the permanence of any such result would depend on securing and maintaining occlusion of the draining bronchus. The procedure was not difficult technically and at first excited considerable interest but after this outburst of enthusiasm transpleural suction drainage of cavities was generally assessed as a method of little intrinsic merit, other than as an occasional preliminary to a thoracoplasty operation and even for that purpose its use was short-lived.

Thoracoplasty. While the surgeons had been collaborating willingly in the physicians' game of ringing the changes on pneumothorax, phrenic paralysis and pneumoperitoneum they had also been devoting considerable time and attention to the operation of thoracoplasty. This was major surgery with a vengeance, not to be embarked on lightly but well worth considering when all else appeared to have failed and when a surgeon with the requisite skill and experience was available. That this latter requirement constituted a problem is apparent in a comment by Christopher Rolleston quoted in the Medical Research Council's Report on Artificial Pneumothorax in 1922.

> Recently in Norway and other continental countries, those cases in which there is obliteration of the pleural cavity by adhesions have been treated by excision of all the ribs on the affected side. Excellent results are reported but it is difficult to find a surgeon in this country to undertake the work.[29]

28 Monaldi, V. (1938) Quoted by Maxwell, R. J. C. & Kohnstamn, M. L. (27).
29 Burrell, L. S. T. & Macnalty, A. S. (2) p. 81.

On the Continent the possibilities of thoracoplasty had been assessed much more rapidly than in Britain. In Germany, Sauerbruch had now taken the lead, had developed the paravertebral thoracoplasty from the work begun by Wilms and was shortly to become the acknowledged master in the field of thoracic surgery. Ferdinand Sauerbruch was born in Barmen in 1875, the son of the manager of a textile factory who died in 1877 from acute tuberculosis. As far as can be gathered from his autobiography, he had no compelling urge to study medicine and teaching had been his first choice. He gave no definite reason for his switch to medicine but stated with much emphasis that he had never regretted the change. He studied at Leipzig where he qualified in 1901 and shortly afterwards, influenced by his experiences with a patient who had been gored by a bull and suffered a pneumothorax, he decided to direct his main attention to 'the physical conditions prevailing within the human thorax'.[30]

Stimulated and encouraged by the interest taken in his researches by his great chief, von Mikulicz, Sauerbruch first of all devised a low pressure chamber, which could accommodate two surgeons and a patient, for use in intrathoracic surgery. In this way he eliminated the immediate lung collapse which otherwise followed when the thorax was opened to atmospheric pressure and, with the aid of this chamber, von Mikulicz himself, assisted by Sauerbruch, performed successfully an operation for the removal of a mediastinal tumour. Thereafter promotion readily came his way and when he accepted the chair of surgery at Zurich, conveniently adjacent to the famous sanatoria of Davos, his explorations into the surgery of pulmonary tuberculosis began. He was later to become professor of surgery at Munich and finally, in 1927, at Berlin when he was at the height of his powers and a world figure in surgical circles. Regrettably he delayed the writing of his autobiography until a year or two before his death when his critical faculties were impaired by the ravages of arteriosclerosis and he elected also to write for a predominantly lay readership. These two factors contributed to the production of a highly dramatized account of his own achievements with much 'name-dropping' as he told of the distinguished international clientele who appeared to flock daily to his consulting room from every corner of Europe. This ill-conceived volume has created a false image of its subject who, although acknowledged even by his admirers to have been dictatorial and arrogant, was nevertheless a great surgeon and a notable pioneer.

30   Sauerbruch, F. (1953) *A Surgeon's Life*. p. 33. London: A. Deutsch.

In his hands the operation of thoracoplasty took effective shape: he realized that while the Brauer–Friedrich operation was too extensive, that which had been evolved by Wilms was not extensive enough. Gradually the typical paravertebral thoracoplasty was developed and it became accepted doctrine that the desired immobilization of the lung could only be made possible by the excision of segments of all the ribs from the first down to the eleventh. This drastic assault on the thoracic cage was carried out in one or, at the most, two stages at the Sauerbruch clinic and also at the other European clinics where the Master's lead was to be followed. It was attended by a fearsome operative mortality varying from the 10 per cent recorded by Bull[31] to the 40.1 per cent reported by Jacobaeus and Key[32] with a 'cure' rate of 34 and 36.6 per cent respectively. Both sets of figures left much room for improvement and, in 1928, Graf in Germany and John Alexander in the United States, working independently, began to remove much greater lengths of the upper ribs, a variation which, they hoped, would bring about a higher rate of cavity closure and consequently of clinical cure. In the same year Alexander took a further step forward when he incorporated into his clinical practice a suggestion which he had put forward in 1925 and forsook the 11-rib Wilms–Sauerbruch operation for a partial thoracoplasty which involved usually the upper seven ribs only. The results in terms of reduced mortality and increased clinical benefit were impressive and Alexander wrote in 1937:

> A partial thoracoplasty in multiple stages of greater lengths of the upper most ribs and of such lengths and numbers of the next lower ribs as the individual patient requires, has become the modern type of thoracoplasty.[33]

The name of John Alexander was held in high regard in American thoracic surgical circles and he was particularly well-known for his interest in the surgery of pulmonary tuberculosis. A native of Philadelphia, he had graduated in medicine in 1916 from the University of Pennsylvania after a distinguished undergraduate career. He served in France with the Medical Corps of the United States Army during World War I and, before returning home, spent a short period in

31 Bull, P. (1924) Ninety-three cases of extrapleural thoracoplasty. *Proc. R. Soc. Med.* *17*, 1.

32 Jacobaeus, H. C. & Key, E. Quoted by Alexander, J. (1937) *The Collapse Therapy of Pulmonary Tuberculosis*. p. 451. Springfield, Illinois: C. C. Thomas.

33 Alexander, J. (32) p. 453.

Lyons with Leon Bérard whose clinic was then employing surgery in the treatment of tuberculosis, an experience which appeared to play a significant part in deciding John Alexander's future interest. He returned for a year to his old university as assistant to the professor of clincial surgery and in 1920 moved to the University of Michigan as instructor in surgery. Shortly afterwards he developed spinal tuberculosis, a set back which unleashed hidden reserves of courage and determination, for, during his enforced sojourn at Saranac Lake, he designed and produced a special support for books which enabled them to be held above the head for the recumbent reader.[34] During this same period he wrote the first of his text books, *The Surgery of Pulmonary Tuberculosis*, in which he summarized the results of others in this new field and in so writing gained the quinquennial Samuel D. Gross Prize of the Philadelphia Academy of Surgery. In 1926 he returned to the University of Michigan and from 1928 onwards he devoted his time and attention almost exclusively to the new speciality of thoracic surgery, publishing in 1937 his classic text *The Collapse Therapy of Pulmonary Tuberculosis*.

John Alexander was not only a skilful surgeon and an inspiring teacher but was also the possessor of a charm of manner which earned him the affection as well as the respect and admiration of all who knew him. He trained more thoracic surgeons than any other teacher of his era and it was these erstwhile trainees who, after his death in 1954, were responsible for the writing and publication of the John Alexander Monograph Series on various aspects of thoracic surgery, dedicated to his memory 'with the affection, admiration and gratitude of the thoracic surgeons whom he trained'.

As far as the United States was concerned the Alexander partial thoracoplasty had come to stay, as was inevitable when the credentials of its progenitor are considered, but there were others elsewhere who were not so satisfied among them being that remarkable pioneer and later doyen of British thoracic surgery, Hugh Morriston Davies. A graduate of Cambridge and of University College Hospital, he qualified in 1903, became a Fellow of the Royal College of Surgeons in 1906 and in 1908 was appointed to the staff of his old teaching hospital. By this time he had decided to make surgery of the chest his special interest and in pursuance of that decision he travelled to Berlin for the Surgical Congress of 1910. There he heard Brauer, Friedrich,

34 Alexander, J. (1926) Reading and writing for the recumbent. *J. Am. med. Ass. 86*, 346.

Wilms and Sauerbruch deliver their epoch-making papers and he came home filled with enthusiasm and determination. Obtaining a small research room in the basement of the hospital he immediately became absorbed in a study of pulmonary disease, utilizing the new methods and techniques of radiology in spite of 'the emphatic assertion of almost everyone that radiographs of the chest were useless in diagnosis'.[35]

Between 1912 and 1915 he carried out a few thoracoplasty operations using the Wilms' technique but in 1916 disaster struck when, during the performance of a rib resection for empyema, a splinter of glass pierced the skin of his right hand. A devastating infection followed and although amputation, which at one stage had appeared inevitable, was avoided he was left with a contracted right hand, the fingers of which were rigidly flexed, distorted and useless. Resigning his surgical appointment he prepared to devote himself to the less physically arduous practice of medicine and, still fascinated by diseases of the chest, he purchased a private sanatorium in the Vale of Clwyd in North Wales in 1918. But the lure of the operating theatre proved irresistible and in 1921 he embarked again on major surgery, operating with his left hand and to such effect that the Vale of Clwyd sanatorium grew into a thoracic centre of note, attracting surgeons from all over the world. By 1924 he had performed 20 thoracoplasty operations for tuberculosis, removing 'portions of the posterior ends of the first ten or eleven ribs through a paravertebral incision' and he was able to report that seven of the patients subsequently became free from symptoms while a further five were 'considerably improved'.[36]

A few years later a visit from John Alexander persuaded him into resecting greater lengths of rib in multiple stages and

As a result many of my thoracoplasty collapses from 1931 to 1935 were so indifferent and even bad that I was tempted to abandon operating. I went to America in 1935 and found their results no better . . . I remodelled my operation removing the whole first and second ribs and 10 to 12 cm only of the rest. In addition I resected the transverse processes to abolish the costo-transverse process-vertebral gutter. The operation was done in two, sometimes three, stages.[37]

Davies remained faithful to this technique throughout his long career and proved completely resistant even to those later modifications of

35 Davies, H. M. (1948) A provocative talk on pulmonary tuberculosis. *Thorax 3*, 189.
36 Davies, H. M. (3).
37 Davies, H. M. (35).

thoracoplasty which, in the eyes of many, changed the character of the operation and brought it truly into modern times.

Thoracoplasty as performed up until 1934 had depended for its effects entirely on the resection of ribs. This permitted only a lateral relaxation of the lung and left the apex, the most usual site for disease, still attached to the thoracic dome and subject to vertical stresses exerted through the scalene muscles above and, to a lesser extent, through the diaphragm below. In such circumstances an upper lobe cavity, although it might be reduced in shape and size to a vertical slit, could still remain patent after operation, a defect that led to many of the failures of thoracoplasty.

Holst and Semb, working in Oslo, had given thought to this problem and had concluded that the ideal thoracoplasty must be capable of producing the same degree and type of relaxation as that achieved by a perfect, adhesion-free pneumothorax—in short, that a concentric relaxation should if possible replace the purely lateral effect obtained by the standard paravertebral operation.[38]

It fell to Carl Semb to devise the manoeuvre which went a long way towards attaining this ideal when he introduced his thoracoplasty with extrafascial apicolysis. In this the rib resection was combined with mobilization of the lung apex in the extrafascial plane by dissecting it free from all the anatomical attachments which anchored it to the adjacent structures. The procedure required considerable technical skill and patience and extended the operating time but it did produce the desired concentric relaxation and also proved to be more conservative in terms of the number of ribs resected than the operation which it was designed to replace. When Semb published his first account of extrafascial apicolysis in 1935 he was able to report that cavity closure had been attained in over 90 per cent of cases with freedom from bacilli in over 80 per cent, while, provided that no more than six ribs were resected at any one stage, the operative mortality was less than 3 per cent.[39] Colloquially known as the 'Semb strip', this operation completely superseded the paravertebral thoracoplasty in European circles while in Britain, apart from Morriston Davies, it was universally adopted by the leading thoracic surgeons.

It was much less generally acclaimed in the United States, where the

38   Holst, J., Semb, C. & Frimann-Dahl, J. (1935) On the surgical treatment of pulmonary tuberculosis. *Acta chir. scand. 76*, Suppl. 34-7.
39   Semb, C. (1935) Thoracoplasty with extrafascial apicolysis. *Acta chir. scand. 76*, Suppl. 34-7.

majority followed the teaching of John Alexander and, during a visit to that country in 1955, the writer did not see a single patient who had had an extrafascial apicolysis in association with his thoracoplasty. This widespread American neglect of Semb's ingenious innovation rendered the thoracic surgeons of that country particularly receptive to the idea of lung resection in the surgery of tuberculosis and much of the early work in this field was to come from the famous clinics of the United States and to bring to the fore a new galaxy of surgical stars.

Lung Resection. The few sporadic resection operations carried out at the close of the nineteenth century, although one or two had been successful, had served mainly to emphasize the hazardous nature of the undertaking and for nearly 40 years the subject was left in abeyance. It was revived as a serious proposition when, in 1935, Freedlander reported success with a deliberate and intentional lobectomy performed for tuberculosis,[40] followed in 1939 by an account by Jones and Dolley of five patients, two of whom had had lobectomies and the remaining three pneumonectomies.[41]

The hunt was now up and at the meeting of the American Association for Thoracic Surgery at Cleveland in 1940 members were invited to report on any resection operations which they might have carried out for tuberculosis. This blanket invitation yielded a total of 19 pneumonectomies and 31 lobectomies: out of that total there were 16 deaths directly associated with the operation to be set against a further 16 patients who were considered to be 'well'.[42] In the discussion which followed the prevailing mood was one of pessimism and Alexander was almost certainly expressing the views of the meeting when he said that accumulating experience showed that resection was very dangerous and only indicated if it was thought that the patient had a greater chance of living if it were done.[43]

But the atmosphere of pessimism was of transient duration only and by 1943 the whole subject was re-opened and given a new lease of life by Churchill and Klopstock, reporting from the Massachusetts General Hospital. Their paper was unique in one important respect:

40 Freedlander, S. O. (1935) Lobectomy in tuberculosis. Report of a case. *J. thorac. Surg. 5,* 132.
41 Jones, J. C. & Dolley, F. S. (1939) Lobectomy and pneumonectomy in pulmonary tuberculosis. *J. thorac. Surg. 8,* 351.
42 Jones, J. C. (1957) *The Surgical Management of Pulmonary Tuberculosis.* (ed. J. D. Steele) p. 26. John Alexander Monograph Series. Springfield, Illinois: C. C. Thomas.
43 *Ibid.* p. 28.

hitherto no surgeon had contemplated resection until all else had failed and now Churchill and his co-author broke new ground by their suggestion that lobectomy be used as 'a highly selective method for dealing with certain unilobar lesions' claiming that it would be more conservative in terms of lung function than either thoraco-plasty or pneumothorax and would also shorten the duration of treatment.[44] This paper represented a turning point in the resection story. Thereafter it was employed with increasing frequency and by 1947 several large series had been reported, including 200 patients operated on by R. H. Overholt, but the price was high with the morbidity rate ranging from 41 to 70 per cent and the mortality rate from 25 to 33 per cent.[45]

This, however, preceded the clinical use of streptomycin which was now about to transform the usefulness of resection surgery and, when streptomycin was reinforced by *para*-aminosalicylic acid and by isoniazid, resection became the first choice among the various operative procedures. Its position as first choice was strengthened by the attention which was by then being increasingly paid to broncho-pulmonary anatomy, the ramifications of which were so beautifully elucidated by R. C. Brock working at the Brompton Hospital,[46] work that led surgeons to think in terms of the pulmonary segments rather than of the lobes. J. M. Chamberlain, regarded as the pioneer of seg-mental resection for tuberculosis, recognized that modern radio-graphic techniques had shown that chronic pulmonary tuberculosis was localized mainly in three pulmonary segments, the apical and posterior segments of the upper lobe and the apical (superior) seg-ment of the lower lobe.[47] Edgar Medlar, working in the pathology department of Bellevue Hospital, New York, and charting the location of post-primary tuberculosis in 96 persons who had died suddenly and unexpectedly, confirmed Chamberlain's ideas.[48] These findings in-augurated a more conservative approach to resection surgery in which, whenever possible, the segment rather than the lobe became the target. Operation was both preceded and accompanied by a course

44 Churchill, E. D. & Klopstock, R. (1943) Lobectomy for pulmonary tuberculosis. *Ann. Surg. 117*, 641.
45 Jones, J. C. (42) p. 29.
46 Brock, R. C. (1946) *The Anatomy of the Bronchial Tree*. London: Oxford University Press.
47 Chamberlain, J. M., Storey, C. F., Klopstock, R. & Daniels, C. F. (1953) Segmental resection for pulmonary tuberculosis (300 cases). *J. thorac. Surg. 26*, 471.
48 Medlar, E. M. (1947) Incidence of tuberculous pulmonary cavities in unexpected deaths investigated at necropsy. *Archs intern. Med. 8*, 407.

of antituberculosis chemotherapy which produced a startling decrease in subsequent complications and, with its aid, what had been a dangerous surgical procedure was converted into a safer, less undesirable and more successful operation, conservative in its approach, and replacing completely the multiple-staged, deforming operations of the immediate past.

In 1956 John D. Steele reported a large series of segmental resections from the Veterans Administration hospitals of the United States with a 1 per cent mortality and a high percentage of cures[49] while in 1958 Brewer and Bai published details of a series of 129 private patients who had had segmental resections with a recovery rate of 98 per cent and a mortality of 0.9 per cent.[50]

In the flush of enthusiasm generated by such reports and figures it was difficult for thoracic surgeons to appreciate that the surgery of pulmonary tuberculosis had outlived its usefulness and that everything which their ingenuity had devised and their skill accomplished was about to be swept away by the rising tide of combined chemotherapy. Yet a completely new era was just upon them: by 1955 collapse therapy had given way to resection surgery and by 1958 resection had in its turn been replaced by long-term chemotherapy and had vanished, never to return.

49   Steele, J. D. (1956) U.S. Veterans Administration—Armed Forces Cooperative Studies of Tuberculosis. IV. Results of pulmonary resection. 1952–55. *Amer. Rev. Tuberc. 73*, 960.

50   Brewer, L. A. & Bai, A. F. (1955) *The Surgical Management of Pulmonary Tuberculosis.* (ed. Sloan, H. & Mines, R.) p. 43. John Alexander Monograph Series. Springfield, Illinois: C. C. Thomas.

Chapter Fifteen
Social and Epidemiological Progress in Tuberculosis Control

While the literature of the earlier part of the twentieth century is liberally studded with the names of those who made contributions, major or minor, to the treatment of the individual case of tuberculosis it contains signally fewer references to pioneer work which was taking place in the field of prevention. The glare of publicity appeared to be dimmed to a faint glow when it was switched from the tensions of the ward and the operating theatre to the more mundane proceedings at the dispensary yet, despite this outward evidence of disinterest, notable discoveries were being made by notable men whose names and records are now seen to shine just as brightly, if not with an even greater intensity, as those of the clinicians.

At the beginning of the century interest was still centred on tuberculin which, despite its dismal failure in therapeutics, had retained untarnished its reputation as an instrument of diagnosis. Research workers in Germany, France and Denmark had established

> that tuberculin was to furnish veterinary medicine with a marvellous means of detecting tuberculosis in cattle, when neither physical examination nor the presence of bacilli in expectoration or in milk could give the information. Then the clinicians who were experimenting with tuberculin on a large scale from a therapeutic point of view and meeting with cruel disappointments, came to realise that this valuable substance was to be used indeed more advantageously for the diagnosis of incipient or doubtful cases of tuberculous infection.[1]

But to enable the diagnostic possibilities of tuberculin to be exploited to the full it was essential to find a safe, painless and reliable means of administration as an alternative to subcutaneous injection

---

1 Calmette, A. (1923) *Tubercle Bacillus Infection and Tuberculosis in Man and Animals.* p. 500 (English trans. by W. B. Soper and G. H. Smith) Baltimore: Williams & Wilkins.

the route originally employed, which was certainly neither painless nor free from risk. The fierce general reaction which signified a positive result was not only an unpleasant experience in itself but was accompanied by focal reactions which 'all too frequently whip up the disease and hasten its progress',[2] disadvantages which rendered the method quite unsuitable for routine diagnostic use. Rectal administration in an enema containing 0.01 g of tuberculin in 50 ml of milk was tried but was found to have disadvantages similar to the subcutaneous route, while a conjunctival test, introduced by Calmette and Wolff-Eisner, working independently,[3] was held to be not only unreliable in its results but unjustifiably painful in its application and was rapidly discarded.[4] The practical problem of tuberculin testing was largely solved through the work of Clemens von Pirquet who, as early as 1903, had advanced the hypothesis that the reaction of tuberculosis to tuberculin was a sensitization phenomenon to which he applied the term *allergy*. Thereafter he embarked on the series of studies which led him in 1907 to the discovery of his cutaneous tuberculin reaction and the development of the simple test which bears his name.[5] The introduction of the von Pirquet test constituted a milestone in the history of tuberculosis though its full significance was not at first appreciated. A distinguished American physician, Allen K. Krause, was later to put the record straight when he wrote in 1919:

> Our awakening began almost so gently that most of us refused to be stirred up. We may date the dawn of this new day to the Pirquet test. This simple manoeuvre, innocently put forward to aid us in diagnosis, to detect the consumptive even before he is aware of impending trouble, did not fulfill its original purpose. It did not point out who were tuberculous enough to be treated and who were not; and viewed from this angle it was a failure . . . But never did a failure lead to more significant results! After several years,—after much grist had gone through the mill, it was found that the Pirquet test and all that it may mean had taught us many things that most of us would not have believed a decade before. Indeed, so multiform and far-reaching are its implications that

4 Hart, P D'A. (1932) The value of tuberculin tests in man. *Medical Research Council Special Report Series No. 164.* London: H.M.S.O.
5 von Pirquet, C. (1907) Der diagnostisch Wert der Kutanen Tuberkulin-reaktion bei der Tuberculose des Kindesalters auf Grund von 100 Sektionen. *Wien. klin. Wschr. 20,* 1123.

it is my own opinion that with Laënnec's promulgation of the unity of phthisis, Villemin's discovery of the infectiousness of tubercle and Koch's revelation of the bacillus, it makes up *the* quartet of really great episodes in the history of tuberculosis. And in some respects I consider the era of ideas,—ideas, many of which are still relatively embryonic and formless,—that it ushered in as the greatest of all.[6]

The awakening to which Krause was referring centred on the then commonly held opinion that tuberculous infection and manifest tuberculosis in an adult were almost simultaneous in their occurrence, a point of view which reflected the overwhelming bacteriological bias which Koch and his disciples had imposed upon preventive medicine. von Pirquet's work shattered this simple concept by demonstrating that while a large proportion of those who lived in close association with their fellows harboured the tubercle bacillus, having become infected comparatively early in life, only a small percentage subsequently developed clinical tuberculosis. The disease was not, therefore, the result of a straightforward bacillus–host relationship but other factors, of which there might well be a multiplicity, would appear to be involved. This surmise was subsequently confirmed as the science of epidemiology came of age and the systematic investigation of the environmental, sociological and immunological variations which could influence the course and outcome of tuberculous infection was begun.

Whilst the credit for the breakthrough inaugurated by his test belongs undisputedly to von Pirquet he was not left long in sole possession of the arena. In the following year Charles Mantoux introduced his intracutaneous test[7] which, although somewhat more elaborate in its technique than von Pirquet's, had an advantage in that the amount of tuberculin required to produce a reaction could be accurately measured. In addition, for the intracutaneous test, the tuberculin was introduced at a known depth in the skin and these two factors endowed it with a superior degree of accuracy as well as comparability when the results of successive tests were being assessed.

In search for the ultimate in simplicity a percutaneous test was devised by Moro.[8] This merely involved direct inunction of the skin with an ointment consisting of 50 per cent old tuberculin in lanolin

6 Krause, A. K. (1919) Antituberculosis measures. *Am. Rev. Tuberc. 2*, 637.
7 Mantoux, C. (1910) L'intradermo-réaction à la tuberculine et son interpretation clinique. *Presse méd., 18*, 10.
8 Moro, E. (1908) Über eine diagnostisch verwertbare Reaktion der Haut auf Einreibung mit Tuberculinsalbe. *Münch med. Wschr., 52*, 216.

but it proved unreliable in practice and, despite its undoubted convenience, failed to gain any measure of acceptance. It may, however, be regarded as the precursor of the tuberculin jelly test and the Vollmer patch test which later proved to be convenient in specific situations where speed and simplicity were of the essence.

Both the von Pirquet and the Mantoux tests were widely used with the Scandinavian countries in particular showing a preference for von Pirquet until, in 1932, the British Medical Research Council came down firmly in favour of the Mantoux test. The latter thereafter gradually forged ahead until, in the 1950s it was challenged but never entirely replaced by the multiple puncture test of Heaf.

A further notable modification in the technique of tuberculin testing was the gradual replacement of old Tuberculin, the original test medium, by a purified protein derivative (PPD) which had been prepared by Esmond R. Long and Florence Seibert in the course of studies carried out mainly at the Henry Phipps Institute in Philadelphia.[9] This substance had the dual advantage both of reducing the non-specific reactions associated with Old Tuberculin and, since it could be prepared with a high degree of uniformity, of ensuring that the results of surveys in which different batches of PPD had been employed could be accurately compared. It was used extensively in projects carried out under the auspices of the World Health Organisation, and in Britain it became the official preparation issued by the Ministry of Health for the tuberculin testing required in association with the BCG campaign.

This is, however, anticipating events. Stepping back again into the earlier decades of the century it becomes clear that the powerful weapon which von Pirquet and Mantoux had placed in the hands of the physicians was having a mixed reception. The accuracy of the information which the tuberculin test could provide was not directly challenged but the interest and enthusiasm with which this information was sought seemed rather patchily distributed. The fact that in 1932 the British Medical Research Council had felt it desirable to support an investigation into the value of tuberculin tests in man suggests that in the United Kingdom these had been somewhat sluggishly applied, a suspicion which is confirmed by the preface to the Council's report which read: 'As the years have moved on tuber-

9 Seibert, F. B. (1941) The history of the development of purified protein derivative tuberculin. *Am. Rev. Tuberc.*, *44*, 1.

culin seems to have been used less rather than more, either for treatment or for diagnosis, by clinicians in Britain'.[10] It is notable also that
of the 346 references quoted in the text of the report fewer than 50 are
from British sources. On the Continent more interest was displayed
and tuberculin surveys had been carried out in most countries. In the
larger European cities it had been noted that the ratio of positive
reactors varied from 10 per cent under one year to 85 per cent between
the ages of 10 to 15 years while from the age of 15 upwards practically
90 per cent gave positive results. One particularly striking observation
was made by Overland who, surveying the dwellers in a village in an
isolated valley in Norway where no fatal case of tuberculosis had
ever been recorded, nevertheless found that 54 per cent of the
inhabitants were positive reactors. The village cattle having been
carefully checked and found to be tuberculin-negative the source of
the infection was ultimately traced to two itinerant tuberculous
school teachers who had visited the hamlet.[11]

While the tuberculin test was proving to be the most effective
instrument so far devised for assessing the incidence of infection in
any given community the clinicians were battling grimly with another
problem which, in default of a solution, was endangering the whole
programme of prevention. W. H. Frost the American epidemiologist,
writing in 1937, listed in order of importance the main activities
which were essential in any such programme:

1. The isolation in sanatoria of *all known* open cases of pulmonary
   tuberculosis, continuing isolation so long as the cases remain open.
2. Adequate medical care, preferably in institutions, for the *known* cases
   of tuberculosis which are active but not in an open stage, since these
   cases constitute the group most likely in the immediate future to
   become infectious.
3. More vigorous effort to find cases of tuberculosis earlier and to bring
   them more promptly under medical care and under isolation if they
   are discharging bacilli.
4. Special protection, including medical observation and advice, and
   financial aid as needed, for those groups who, though not at the time
   suffering from tuberculosis, are most imminently endangered.[12]

10 Hart, P.D'A. (4).
11 Baldwin, E. R., Petroff S. A. & Gardner, L. U. (1927) *Tuberculosis. Bacteriology,
Pathology and Laboratory Diagnosis.* p. 213. London: Baillière, Tindall & Cox.
12 Frost, W. H. (1937) How much control of tuberculosis? *Am. J. Pub. Health* 27, 759.

Frost's recommendations were admirable but, unfortunately, there was one major impediment to their implementation. The early diagnosis of clinical tuberculosis was proving an almost unattainable ideal. Compulsory notification—which, at the time of its introduction, had been regarded by some ebullient optimists as the key to the rapid elimination of tuberculosis as a significant cause of death—was not fulfilling expectations. Kingston Fowler described it as 'one of several weak links in the administrative chain which holds in check the natural tendency of the disease to increase the number of its victims'[13] and justified his description by reference to the Ministry of Health Report for 1920 which recorded that in many areas a large proportion of the notified cases were in a very late stage of the disease at the time of notification, while in a not inconsiderable number of instances notification did not reach the Medical Officer of Health until after the death of the patient. Commenting on the greatly increased opportunities for the spread of infection which arose from this situation, Fowler called it 'a serious blot on the efficiency of the Tuberculosis Service'—a judgment which was in the circumstances somewhat harsh and suggested an over-simplification of a complex problem to which many factors were contributing. Prominent amongst these was the acknowledged fact that the symptoms associated with the onset of tuberculosis were so vague, insidious and non-specific that the victim, unless he was unduly prone to introspection, failed to recognize that they indicated a departure from the normal until the disease had gained a firm grip. Even when advice was sought in the early symptomatic stage a correct diagnosis did not necessarily follow, for few dispensaries of that period possessed X-ray equipment and the physical signs on which reliance had to be placed were either absent or so slight as to escape detection.

One further and very important deterrent which restrained many from seeking advice until serious symptoms had intervened was the undoubted economic hardship which treatment for tuberculosis imposed upon its victim and his family. Even in the late 1930s, when greater enlightenment might have been anticipated, this economic stress remained severe. Sickness benefit from National Health Insurance funds was payable only for six months, after which it was replaced by National Health Insurance disablement which was not

13 Fowler, J. Kingston (1923) *Problems in Tuberculosis.* p. 34. London: Frowde & Hodder & Stoughton.

only inadequate for the patients' own needs but made no provision for his family. In the circumstances it is hardly an exaggeration to say that to undergo treatment for tuberculosis meant a descent into impoverishment and hence to the patient the dispensary all too frequently became a court of last resort.

This was the situation pertaining at the outbreak of World War II except that by then the majority of dispensaries had been equipped with X-ray departments and adequate provision had been made for sanatorium treatment but in spite of these improvements the Chief Medical Officer to the Ministry of Health found it still necessary to write in his annual report for 1939 that 'it is to be regretted that the figures do not give any indication that a greater number of persons are diagnosed in the earlier stages of the disease'.[14]

The fire and enthusiasm which had been so evident at the initiation of the campaign for prevention appeared to have been damped down. It seemed as though the health authorities, intimidated by the daunting nature and complexity of their task, were drawing comfort from the researches of Brownlee who, employing mortality records as the basis for his work, had established the epidemic nature of tuberculosis.[15] His figures showed that in London the epidemic had appeared to reach its peak about 1801 when phthisis accounted for 30 per cent of the total deaths after which it fell gradually until by 1910 it had reached 9 per cent, eliciting from Brownlee the comment that 'the epidemic of phthisis is coming to an end the course of which apparently has been something like two hundred years'.

In the United States, Drolet, studying three large centres of population, had demonstrated a somewhat similar pattern, showing a steady decline in death rate from 1880 when the figure was about 300 deaths per 100 000 of population until 1935 when a figure of 69 per 100 000 was reached.[16] Findings such as these were an encouragement to health authorities to believe that by merely holding the fort and refraining from costly forays outwith its defences nature and the natural history of epidemics would eventually combine to resolve their difficulties and it is notable that about this period there was a

---

14   Ministry of Health (1939) *Report of the Chief Medical Officer.* p. 29. London: H.M.S.O.
15   Brownlee, J. (1918, 1920) An investigation into the epidemiology of phthisis in Great Britain and Ireland. *Special Report Series Nos 18 and 46*. London: H.M.S.O.
16   Drolet, G. (1939) *Clinical Tuberculosis.* (ed. by B. Goldberg) p. A4. Philadelphia: Davis.

significant change in nomenclature with the replacement of 'prevention' by the less ambitious term 'control'. So health authorities everywhere pressed on with examination of contacts, created more sanatorium beds, issued routine pleas for earlier diagnosis and generally coasted along with their problem until the pressures of World War II shattered their hopes and galvanized them into taking new and decisive action which revitalized the whole campaign.

The impact of the war upon tuberculosis trends in Britain was immediate and the decline in mortality which had been taking place gradually during the pre-war years was not only halted abruptly but was actually reversed, the reversal involving both respiratory and non-respiratory forms. An increase in mortality was noted in 1940 with a further increase in 1941 in which year deaths from respiratory tuberculosis alone showed a rise of 10 per cent in England and Wales and of 18 per cent in Scotland compared with the average of the pre-war years of 1938 and 1939. A further cause for concern was a sharp rise in deaths from meningeal tuberculosis, affecting all age groups up to 45.

Acutely alarmed, the Ministry of Health appointed in 1941, under the auspices of the Medical Research Council, a Committee on Tuberculosis in War-Time with the following terms of reference:

> To assist in promoting an investigation of the extent and causes of the war-time increase in the incidence of tuberculosis, particularly among young women, and also to advise the Council regarding possible preventive measures.

The Committee submitted its report in September 1942.[17] In this document stress was laid upon the importance, as causative factors, of certain circumstances peculiar to World War II of which the following were the most important. The government policy of evacuating tuberculosis hospitals and sanatoria in September 1939 to make way for a feared inrush of air raid casualties had resulted in the return of a large number of infectious cases to their homes, while blackout conditions in the home and in the factory had impaired ventilation, increased cross-infection and lowered resistance. The increase in cases of non-respiratory disease was believed to be linked to the large-scale evacuation of town-bred children, who normally

17 Medical Research Council (1942) *Report of Committee on Tuberculosis in War-Time* London: H.M.S.O.

consumed pasteurized milk, to country areas where they had to change to raw milk in the absence of pasteurizing facilities.

After rightly drawing attention to the highly unsatisfactory nature of the national milk supply *vis à vis* tuberculosis and pressing for a massive extension of pasteurization, the Committee made a number of other recommendations, two of which were of outstanding importance. The first, an attempt to eliminate the danger of infection from unsuspected cases as well as to improve the prognosis for the individual sufferer, concentrated on the age-old problem of early diagnosis and advised that the initiative for X-ray examination should now pass from patient to doctor, a solution which had been made possible by the timely development of mass radiography. Since resources in 1942 did not permit any extravagant use of this facility the Committee recommended that initially the available apparatus should be concentrated on those groups in which, either through the nature of the employment or the composition of those at risk, a relatively high incidence of pulmonary tuberculosis might be expected, adding that 'It would favour the introduction of further schemes in the industrial population as soon as the supply of apparatus makes this practicable'.

The second outstanding recommendation was that some form of additional financial help should be provided which, by easing the economic consequences of diagnosis, might encourage the patient to seek treatment earlier. The Committee suggested that such financial provision should ensure an adequate allowance for up to one year after notification, the amount to vary according to the needs of the patient and his family, while at the expiry of the one year period the case could be reviewed and the amount of the allowance adjusted to meet the prevailing circumstances.

The fact that both these recommendations were accepted by the Ministry of Health and subsequently implemented is a fairly accurate reflection of the very considerable degree of public concern which the increase in tuberculosis evoked. It is true that the proposed financial benefits, outlined in an official document Memo 266/T(1943), were initially on a limited scale but even if they appeared lacking in generosity in the beginning, the essential breakthrough had been achieved and more realistic financial provision for the tuberculous patient and his dependants was to follow in succeeding years when the benefits of the scheme had proved themselves beyond any denial.

Mass miniature radiography was rapidly recognized as one of the major innovations of the century since, by the 1930s, it had become clear to all what the more perspicacious had been saying for years, namely that a radiograph of the chest was superior to any other method of examination for the detection of tuberculosis with accuracy and certainty in either its pre-clinical or early clinical phase. It appeared to be a method which could be adapted to large scale studies and its possibilities in this respect had already been explored in limited surveys when standard films had been employed.[18] To continue the use of standard films for extensive community studies would, unfortunately, have proved a prohibitively expensive exercise so two other possibilities were considered. The first, employing cheaper photographic paper instead of film, gave results which were technically less satisfactory, was equally time-consuming and provided a storage problem, while the second, examination by fluoroscopic screen alone, was inhibited by the triple handicap of early observer-fatigue with consequent sacrifice of accuracy, lack of any permanent record and an appreciable radiation risk.

All these difficulties were to be triumphantly overcome by the introduction of miniature radiography which consisted quite simply of miniature photography of the chest image as shown on the fluorescent screen. The idea was not the result of a sudden inspiration or flash of genius on the part of any single individual for a number of workers in various countries had been experimenting along these lines from the very year of Röntgen's original discovery.[19, 20] For a time the technical problems proved unsurmountable but during the decade 1925 to 1935 these difficulties were resolved and mass miniature radiography was transformed from a possibility into a reality, thus providing health authorities everywhere with a rapid, inexpensive, mobile and accurate diagnostic service. The production of the various items required for the finished product was a truly international effort: Holland invented the fine focus rotating anode tube, Britain produced the highly luminescent Levy West screen, Germany was responsible for the wide aperture lens, while America, Britain and Germany all developed the requisite fine-grain, fast film. It remained for a Brazilian physician to put all these together and to

18   British Tuberculosis Association (1940) Detection of early tuberculosis. *Br. med. J.* *1*, 361.
19   Caldwell, E. W. (1911) Photography of the fluorescent screen for Röntgen kinematography and other purposes *Am. Q. Roentg. 3*, 34.
20   Bentley, F. J. & Leitner, Z. A. (1940) Mass radiography with special reference to screen photography and pulmonary tuberculosis. *Br. med. J., 1*, 879.

make a fundamental contribution to preventive medicine by his inauguration of the first ever mass miniature radiography or, as he termed it, collective fluorography, service in the world.

Manoel de Abreu had come from Rio de Janeiro during World War I to study in the hospitals of Paris where he first tackled the problem of miniature radiography in 1918. He reverted to it again in 1924 but on neither occasion did he meet with any success. Endowed with persistence and with complete confidence in the ultimate feasibility of the project he pressed on with his researches, taking advantage of each technical development as it came to hand, and eventually he was able to write:

> We inaugurated the first installation of fluorographic apparatus for the purpose of carrying out a collective thoracic survey at the German Hospital of Rio de Janeiro in 1936; thus our priority cannot be contested.[21]

By 1937 a further three centres were operating and early in 1939 he was able to record that

> due to the great interest aroused by this work, we have 25 installations in Brazil and many others in Argentine, Chile, Uruguay, Germany, France etc. The method has also been carried to the United States by Dr. D. O. N. Lindbert . . . Today, three years after the first practical results were achieved, collective fluorography is universally accepted.[22]

Apart from the inevitable few murmurs from the chronic dissenters and from the obtuse who invariably regarded every new idea as unworkable, the introduction of mass miniature radiography was notably free from controversy. In Britain, its endorsement by the Medical Research Council's Committee having been accepted by the Ministry of Health without delay or demur, an official announcement was made in December 1942 to the effect that mobile miniature radiography sets would be made available for the use of a limited number of local authorities, the limits being set only by the restrictions on production and staffing imposed by war conditions. By 1945, 13 local authorities were operating the scheme and the Medical Research Council had issued a report on the *Mass Miniature Radiography of Civilians for the Detection of Pulmonary Tuberculosis* which embodied advice on administrative procedure and technique in operating a

21 de Abreu, M. (1939) Collective fluorography. *Radiology. 33*, 363.
22 *Ibid.*

35 mm mobile apparatus.[23] The build-up continued; in 1949 there were 22 centres throughout Britain providing mass radiography services[24] and by the end of 1950 5 777 637 persons in England and Wales had been radiographed. Of these 3.7 per 1000 were found to have unsuspected active tuberculosis.[25]

With the introduction of mass radiography and of special financial allowances for tuberculosis patients the situation of stalemate which had existed for years appeared to have been broken. A new spirit of endeavour and even of optimism became apparent in the ranks of the Service which received a further boost to its morale and opportunities when the introduction of the National Health Service in 1948 removed specialist medical services from local authority to regional control. Thereafter closer links were forged between the tuberculosis service and general medicine and surgery, thus undoing the harm engendered by the original decisions of the Astor Report in 1912 and leaving personnel of the tuberculosis service poised to embrace with energy and enthusiasm the era of chemotherapy which almost overnight was to change the thinking of the centuries.

23   Medical Research Council (1945) *Mass Miniature Radiography of Civilians*. London: H.M.S.O.
24   McDougall, J. B. (1949) *Tuberculosis. A global study in social pathology*. p. 285. Edinburgh: E. & S. Livingstone.
25   Pagel, W., Simmonds F. A. H., Macdonald N. & Nassau E. (1964) *Pulmonary Tuberculosis* p. 469. London: Oxford University Press.

Chapter Sixteen
Specific Immunization

With physicians, surgeons, pathologists and epidemiologists all involved in the antituberculosis campaign it was only logical and reasonable that the exponents of immunology should wish to add their contribution to the general armamentarium. The series of events constituting the Koch Phenomenon and demonstration that a guinea-pig which had been infected with tuberculosis became, after a short period, refractory to a second infection, appeared to open up the way for their participation. It was argued that if a prophylactic vaccine were to replace the primary infection then any subsequent invasion by virulent bacilli would meet the same fate as the second infection of the phenomenon, a view which seemed to be supported by Marfan's dictum that those who had had scrofula had less tendency to develop progressive tuberculosis.[1]

A vast amount of ingenious experimental work ensued which has been extensively reviewed by Calmette.[2] Vaccines made from killed bacilli and from live bacilli were tried and abandoned and interest was then directed to the possibility of using either naturally or artificially attenuated strains. An example of the former was Friedmann's vaccine which he prepared from an acid-fast bacillus isolated from turtles, a bacillus which was shown to be devoid of virulence for warm-blooded animals. Unfortunately it proved to be equally devoid of any immunizing properties and was eventually discarded.

The quest continued and persistence was ultimately rewarded through a fortuitous observation. Albert Calmette and his assistant, Camille Guérin, a veterinarian from Limoges, were working at the

1 Marfan, A. B. (1886) De l'immunité conférée par la guérison d'une tuberculose locale pour la phthisie pulmonaire. *Archs. gén. Méd.* *57*, 575.
2 Calmette, A. (123) *Tubercle Bacillus Infection and Tuberculosis in Man & Animals.* pp. 624, 654 (English trans. by W. B. Soper and G. H. Smith) Baltimore: Williams & Wilkins.

Pasteur Institute at Lille using a virulent strain of bovine tubercle bacilli which had been isolated by Nocard from the udder of a tuberculous cow. They were growing this organism on a glycerin-bile-potato medium, a convenient method of obtaining a homo-geneous suspension of the culture in saline, when they noted that repeated subculturing was leading to a progressive loss in virulence.[3] By the time that this observation was made most investigators had come to the conclusion that only a live vaccine could be relied upon to produce immunity and accordingly Calmette and Guérin in 1908 embarked upon an attempt to reduce the virulence of this organism to a point when it might be considered suitable for a vaccination programme.

At the start of the project the virulence of the strain was such that 3 mg, injected intraveneously into a calf, resulted in death from progressive tuberculosis within 28 to 35 days. After approximately 70 subcultures on the glycerin-bile-potato medium the virulence was so far diminished that the animal was able to tolerate the injection of 100 mg, 'without producing the slightest tubercle formation'.[4] Throughout the World War I and even during the period when Lille was occupied by the Germans the patient process of subculturing continued and by 1919 the organism was incapable of producing tuberculosis in guinea pigs, rabbits, horses and cattle.[5] In 1921 Calmette named this strain Bacille Calmette-Guérin (BCG) and in 1924 he declared it to be a 'virus fixe', a new strain of bacilli which would breed true to type in all circumstances.

Even before this pronouncement by Calmette the first step towards the practical application of a policy of immunization based on BCG had been taken in 1921 when B. Weill-Hallé gave an oral vaccine prepared from it to an infant whose mother had died from tuberculosis a few days after its birth. The child maintained good health. Thereafter the use of the vaccine was gradually extended and by 1928 over 116 000 infants had received it in France alone.[6]

Calmette's enthusiasm communicated itself to his fellow country-men but elsewhere the development of BCG was viewed with a certain mistrust. The lack of any controlled experiment excited adverse comment and, in the absence of the evidence which only such an

3 *Ibid.* p. 654.
4 *Ibid.* p. 654.
5 Irvine, K. N. (1949) *BCG Vaccination in Theory and Practice.* p. 4. Oxford: Blackwell.
6 McDougall, J. B. (1949) *Tuberculosis: A Global Study in Social Pathology.* p. 393. Edinburgh: Livingstone.

experiment could provide, many workers outside France opposed
its introduction into their own countries. Such statistical evidence
as Calmette did produce was subjected to severe criticism, a particularly devastating attack being mounted by Greenwood, professor
of epidemiology and vital statistics in the University of London,
who, after enumerating the statistical errors in a publication by
Calmette covering his work from July 1924 to December 1927, stated
that

> he has deliberately appealed to the statistical method, and, in my sub-
> mission, his use of that method has been so grossly defective that no
> confidence can be placed either in his statistical inferences or in the
> reliability of the data which he has assembled. The collection of data is at
> least as delicate a business as their analysis, and a writer who shows so
> little respect for logic in analysis is not likely to have been more cir-
> cumspect in assembling data for analysis.[7]

Immediately following Greenwood's onslaught came another
publication which must have done much to convince the sceptics of
the wisdom of their attitude. In 1929 Petroff, Branch and Steenken,
working in the Research and Clinical Laboratory at the Trudeau
Sanatorium, claimed to have grown a virulent variant from three
separate cultures of BCG, two of which had been supplied from
Calmette's own laboratory.[8] This cast very serious doubt on the claim
that BCG was a 'virus fixe' and Calmette reacted violently and angrily.
Further evidence from other sources appeared to support the views
of Petroff and his colleagues although in assessing much of this
evidence McDougall found it difficult to exclude completely possible
sources of error including contamination of cultures, mistaken
diagnosis of lesions in experimental animals and even cross-infection
in animal houses and added that 'Many excellent workers were,
however, unable to demonstrate any degree of virulence even when
following exactly the technique of workers who had claimed to have
proved the virulence of the strain'.[9] While there was obviously some
conflict of evidence it nevertheless becomes difficult to avoid a
suspicion that the early strains of BCG were not quite the 'virus fixe'

7 Greenwood, M. (1928) Professor Calmette's statistical study of BCG vaccination.
Br. med. J. 1, 793.
8 Petroff, S. A., Branch, A. & Steenken, W. (1929) A study of Bacillus Calmette-Guerin
(BCG) *Am. Rev. Tuberc. 19*, 9.
9 McDougall, J. B. (6) p. 394.

which Calmette claimed but were made up of a mixture of virulent and avirulent forms.

But the controversy which was thus building up around the vaccine was as nothing compared to what lay just ahead, for in 1930 its reputation was dealt what at first must have seemed a mortal blow by the historic disaster at Lübeck. In this north German town 249 babies, all in the first ten days of life, were given oral BCG and in the succeeding months 67 of these infants died from acute tuberculosis. The protagonists of the vaccine were horrified and shattered, the antagonists proclaimed at once that all their doubts and fears had been amply vindicated and in some countries the use of BCG was suspended. The German government immediately instituted a most rigorous enquiry into all the circumstances, appointing Professor Ludwig Lange and Professor Bruno Lange as their official experts while at the same time inviting a number of other well-known German scientists to give evidence regarding their own personal experiences with BCG. The result of the enquiry was to establish beyond all doubt that the tragedy was not due to the BCG but to its contamination by a culture of virulent tubercle bacilli which, issued originally by Professor Bruno Lange's laboratory at the Institut Robert Koch, had been sent to the laboratory at Kiel and thence had found its way to Lübeck where it had been stored in the same incubator as the vaccine.[10] Some of those involved in this glaring breach of elementary precautions were prosecuted and received prison sentences but it has always been believed that the intense anxiety and strain to which Calmette was subjected at this time contributed substantially to his own death in 1933—too soon to savour the vindication and international recognition which his work was ultimately to be accorded.

Despite the exoneration of the BCG strain from any responsibility for Lübeck the idea that the vaccine could still show a dangerous degree of virulence survived amongst those who wished to believe it. BCG was still readily acceptable in France and in the French-speaking countries but it was fairly generally rejected in Germany and in the United States with Britain adopting an attitude of strict neutrality, not condemning the vaccine but waiting patiently for some other country to provide proof of its efficacy and complete safety.

Convincing evidence was shortly to come from Scandinavia

10   Calmette, A. (1931) Epilogue de la catastrophe de Lübeck. *Presse. med. 2*, 17.

where, both in Norway and in Sweden, the prophylactic possibilities of BCG were being steadily explored along much more scientific lines than those followed by the French workers. In Gothenburg Arvid Wallgren had been vaccinating all infants born in tuberculous homes from 1927 onwards. He believed that the oral administration of the vaccine was often stultified by inadequate absorption and he found that its subcutaneous injection was associated with troublesome abscess formation. He therefore discarded both techniques on the grounds that they were likely to bring the vaccine into disrepute and elected to use intradermal injection which proved to be both effective and free from any notable local complications. In the circumstances in which he was working a controlled experiment was not possible but by December 1933 he was able to show a significant and worthwhile reduction in the death-rate from tuberculosis of this vulnerable group of infants and had satisfied himself that BCG vaccination had made an important contribution to this result.[11] In Norway Johannes Heimbeck was engaged in the prolonged study of probationer nurses at Ulleval Hospital from which he was to emerge with impressive figures from a vaccinated group and a control group.[12] Denmark followed the lead given by Norway and Sweden and gradually, over a period of about 20 years, these Scandinavian countries accumulated evidence and built up a scientific argument for the safety and efficacy of BCG which led, in the late 1940s, to a renewal of world interest in the possibilities of successful immunization.

The result of this renewed interest became fully evident at the conclusion of World War II, when the European participants found themselves with a severe tuberculosis problem on their hands. Scandinavian help to deal with this problem began early in 1947 when the Danish Red Cross initiated a programme of mass BCG vaccination in Hungary, Poland and Germany. Subsequently as other European countries, having assessed their own tuberculosis position and concluded that it was greater than their national resources could cope with, appealed for assistance the Swedish Red Cross and the Norwegian Relief for Europe organization joined their Danish colleagues in an extension of the vaccination programme, thus creating the International Tuberculosis Campaign, more familiarly termed the

---

11 Wallgren, A. (1924) Value of Calmette vaccination in prevention of tuberculosis in childhood. *J. Am. med. Ass. 103*, 1341.
12 Heimbeck, J. (1936) Tuberculosis in hospital nurses. *Tubercle. 18*, 97.

Joint Enterprise. The United Nations organization was associated with the Joint Enterprise through its International Children's Emergency Fund (UNICEF), the association and its objectives being defined by the Director of the Joint Enterprise, the Danish physician Johannes Holm, in the following terms:

> The Joint Enterprise is a co-operative effort between UNICEF and the Scandinavian Voluntary Organisations on an international scale, primarily with the object of assisting national health authorities in the execution of mass BCG vaccination campaigns, and in introducing BCG vaccination as one of the tools in their long-range tuberculosis control programme ... The Joint Enterprise was created specifically to administer BCG vaccination. Both parties are convinced that BCG vaccination gives protection against tuberculosis, and are aware that the effect will be appreciable only if the vaccination is administered on a mass scale. Therefore the Joint Enterprise is interested only in *mass vaccination*. In practice this means that the Joint Enterprise does not embark on a campaign unless a country agrees to an overall BCG vaccination campaign.[13]

In Europe, Austria, Czechoslovakia, Finland, Greece, Hungary, Italy, Poland and Yugoslavia all requested assistance and all signified their agreement to a mass campaign—although the Italian health authorities subsequently found that they had underestimated the influence of a vociferous coterie of physicians opposed to BCG and the Italian campaign, with little accomplished, was terminated by the Joint Enterprise on 1 May 1950.[14] By 1 September 1949 about 8000 000 children and young adults in Europe had received BCG and requests for assistance from further afield were reaching the Joint Enterprise headquarters in Copenhagen. Wherever possible these requests were met and by the end of 1950 vaccination campaigns under the aegis of the Joint Enterprise had been inaugurated in North Africa, the Middle East, Ceylon, India, Pakistan and in two countries in Latin America, Ecuador and Mexico.[15]

There was, therefore, a formidable body of opinion throughout the world so strongly convinced of the efficacy of BCG that governments were unhesitatingly committing themselves to mass campaigns. But not *all* governments! In Britain the Ministry of Health sat firmly

13 International Tuberculosis Campaign (1949) *Conference on European BCG Programmes.* p. 33. Copenhagen.
14 International Tuberculosis Campaign (1951) *Second Annual Report.* pp. 178–80. Copenhagen.
15 Ibid. p. 15.

on the fence despite increasing pressure from tuberculosis workers in favour of BCG. A memorandum prepared by Professor W. H. Tytler and incorporating the views of the Joint Tuberculosis Council, the Tuberculosis Association and the National Association for the Prevention of Tuberculosis, all strongly advocating the use of BCG, was presented to the Ministry of Health in 1944.[16] Some two years later, on 17 July 1946, the chief medical officer to the Ministry agreed to receive a deputation representing those associated with the memorandum and thereafter an official statement was issued to the medical press in which the Minister expressed his willingness to see if a suitable preparation of BCG could be made available, adding 'As regards the use to which it should be put and the class of persons to be vaccinated, it would be necessary to appoint an expert committee to take charge of these details.'

But the voice of caution was still to be heard in the land and in 1947 G. S. Wilson, Director of the Public Health Laboratory Service, was expressing the opinion that unless the gain from BCG vaccination was likely to be substantial there was no good reason for its employment in Britain. He considered that any decision to use the vaccine should be preceded by a controlled trial, or should this prove impractical, then its release should only be sanctioned under strictly defined conditions.[17]

In the event the Ministry, acting in conjunction with the Medical Research Council, decided upon a controlled trial of BCG; a Tuberculosis Vaccines Clinical Trials Committee was appointed and ultimately what proved to be one of the most convincing of all trials ever conducted got under way. In it more than 50 000 children, initially free both from active tuberculosis and from known contact with the disease at home, participated and were scrupulously followed up for periods ranging from seven and a half to ten years. When the Trials Committee reported to the Medical Research Council in 1963 it was able to show that the annual incidence of tuberculosis in the vaccinated group was 0.43 per thousand as against 1.91 per thousand in the tuberculin-negative unvaccinated controls. This represented a reduction in incidence of 79 per cent which the Committee considered could be attributed to the protective effect of the

16 Tytler, W. H. (1944) *Memorandum* on BCG. London.
17 Wilson, G. S. (1947) The value of BCG vaccination in control of tuberculosis. *Br. med. J.* 2, 855.

vaccination.[18] It is probably worth noting that, even before this trial began, the highly favourable reports from Scandinavia had led to government sanction being given in 1949 for the vaccination of persons considered to be at special risk—such as nurses, medical students and contacts of tuberculous patients. From 1954 onwards, following favourable preliminary reports from the Trials Committee, most health authorities began the voluntary vaccination of all school leavers at the age of thirteen.

While Europe, North Africa and large areas of Asia were prepared to welcome BCG the situation on the other side of the Atlantic remained vastly different. In Brazil vaccination by the oral route, as originally practised by Calmette, had been used extensively but even though De Assis, one of the acknowledged authorities on the subject, introduced a vaccine containing a very high proportion of BCG organisms [19] much of it appeared lacking in potency and in the absence of convincing evidence as to its reliability it gradually fell into disuse.

In the United States the reception accorded BCG was, from the very outset, heavily tinged with scepticism and suspicion. The Saranac Laboratory report, which had cast doubt on the safety of the vaccine, undoubtedly was a major contributor to the general attitude, while Greenwood's ruthless exposé of the statistical fallacies in Calmette's earlier publications had not passed unnoticed. To add to the confusion two trials of the vaccine within the United States had given conflicting results. In New York Levine and Sackett's group of vaccinated infants had failed to show significantly superior results over a control group chosen by the method of alternative selection.[20] By contrast Aronson and Palmer, in a well-controlled study of BCG in North American Indians, were able to show that the vaccine gave some degree of protection against all types of lesions but particularly against the more serious pulmonary and extrapulmonary manifestations.[21] Although there were loopholes in the trial by Levine and Sackett such conflicting reports, nevertheless, did nothing to resolve

18 Third Report of Clinical Trials Committee to Medical Research Council. (1963) BCG & vole bacillus vaccines in the prevention of tuberculosis in adolescence and early adult life. *Br. med. J. 1*, 973.
19 De Assis, A. (1957) *Advances in Tuberculosis Research. 8*, 105.
20 Levine, M. I. & Sackett, M. F. (1946) Results of BCG immunization in New York City. *Am. Rev. Tuber. 53*, 517.
21 Aronson, J. D. & Palmer, C. E. (1946) Experiences with BCG vaccination in the control of tuberculosis among North American Indians. *Publ. Hlth Reps., Wash. 61*, 802.

the national doubt and the issue was clouded still further by the emergence of an extremely vocal anti-BCG lobby who put their point of view in a publication in the *British Medical Journal* in June 1959.[22] Entitled *The Case against BCG* and bearing the names of seventeen American physicians of varying degrees of distinction, the communication lived up to its title, presenting the 'cons' without any serious attempt to discuss the 'pros' and displaying so much bias as to be self-defeating. In the circumstances it not unnaturally failed to influence British or Continental thinking, but in the United States opinion generally remained unfavourable to BCG* and this antagonism was whipped up still further by the vehement partisanship of J. Arthur Myers of the University of Minnesota. Myers, one of the authors of *The Case against BCG* continued his attack on the vaccine in his book *Tuberculosis and other Communicable Diseases*[5] an attack remarkable for its apparent lack of scientific objectivity and its inadequately supported allegations of the dire sequelae which followed in the wake of BCG.[23]

These remarks might normally have appealed only to the undiscriminating but the results of two trials organized by the United States Public Health Service in Puerto Rico[24] and in the southern states of Georgia and Alabama[25] appeared to indicate that, in these areas at least, the degree of protection conferred by the vaccine was low—a finding which naturally led to hesitancy amongst even the most unbiassed and scientifically orientated American physicians. Carroll Palmer, who had been closely associated with the conduct of both these United States trials, suggested that the discrepancies between their results and those of the British Medical Research Council's trial might be explained by the much greater frequency of non-specific

* The antipathy to BCG displayed in some areas of the United States was often unreasoning and more in the nature of an emotional outburst than an attempt at scientific appraisal. The author recalls being present in 1955 at a discussion on BCG in a centre in a mid-western state which an American particpant opened by defining BCG as 'a substance designed to give a false sense of security to a man with an unwarranted fear of tuberculosis'.

22   Anderson, A. S., Dickey, L. B. *et al.* (1959) The Case against BCG. *Br. med. J. 1*, 1423.
23   Myers, J. A. (1959) *Tuberculosis and Other Communicable Diseases* pp. 25–6. Springfield, Ill: Thomas.
24   Palmer, C. E., Shaw, L. W. & Comstock, G. W. (1958) Community Trials in BCG vaccination. *Am. Rev. resp. Dis. 77*, 877.
25   Comstock, G. W. & Palmer, C. E. (1966) Long-term results of BCG vaccination in the southern United States. *Am. Rev. resp. Dis. 93*, 171.

mycobacterial infection in the American areas[26] coupled with the British selection of a higher dose of tuberculin for the pre-vaccination eligibility test—a hypothesis which would go far towards reconciling the differing findings.

In 1972, at the Annual Meeting of the American Thoracic Society, a communication by Paneth and Speizer appeared to offer a gleam of hope that a more flexible approach to vaccination was imminent. They advocated the use of BCG in the prevention of infant and child-hood tuberculosis pointing out that in the United States 11 per cent of tuberculosis appeared in children under 15 years of age—a pro-portion that was 'three to five times higher than in a sample of European nations that use BCG'[27]—and went on to suggest that this high risk group be vaccinated at birth, adding figures to show that the cost of such a programme of prophylaxis would be con-siderably less than that of other forms of tuberculosis control.

But deeply ingrained prejudices were not to be so readily eradicated and in 1974 the *American Review of Respiratory Disease*, a much respected and generally authoritative journal, extended the hospitality of its editorial columns to a leading article entitled 'Some of the BCG trials and certain aspects involved in them'.[28] The guest writer, a Dr K. Naganna, who described himself as a statistical officer employed in a Tuberculosis Prevention Trial which was taking place in southern India, made use of his editorial freedom to review the various trials which had been conducted elsewhere. He paid special attention to the British Medical Research Council's trial about which he made the somewhat astounding suggestion that 'bias on the part of the in-vestigators as well as in the methods of investigation during the BMRC trial cannot be completely ruled out'. In the correspondence which followed this publication the numerous fallacies readily detectable in Naganna's argument were forcefully underlined. Amongst this correspondence was a letter from Johannes Guld who, commenting on important omissions from the text of the editorial, expressed the opinion that these omissions appeared 'to be wilful misrepresentations of the evidence rather than just due to careless-

---

26 Palmer, C. E. & Long, M. W. (1966) Effects of infection with atypical mycobacteria on BCG vaccination and tuberculosis. *Am. Rev. resp. Dis. 94,* 553.

27 Paneth, N. & Speizer, F. E. (1972) The role of BCG vaccination in the prevention of tuberculosis in the United States. *Am. Rev. resp. Dis. 105,* 1019.

28 Naganna, K. (1974) Some of the BCG trials and certain aspects involved in them. Editorial. *Am. Rev. resp. Dis. 109,* 497.

ness'[29] while the director of the Indian project in which Naganna was employed wrote to dissociate himself and the other members of the project team from the views expressed by their statistical officer.[30]

American opposition, vocal though it was, failed to influence European opinion nor did it shake the unreserved endorsement bestowed upon the vaccine by the World Health Organisation. Nevertheless, once it was realized that effective chemotherapy was well on the way towards drawing the sting of the tubercle bacillus there appeared to be a slackening in the momentum of the BCG campaign. A detailed epidemiological study carried out between 1961 and 1966 and covering centres in France, Poland, Switzerland and Yugoslavia revealed that a disconcertingly high proportion of children had not been vaccinated. Thus in Geneva, where vaccination was *voluntary*, the proportion unvaccinated was 84 per cent while in France, Calmette's native country, where vaccination was *compulsory* 73 per cent had escaped the net. In Poland and Yugoslavia the unvaccinated amounted to 51 per cent and 24 per cent respectively.[31] This investigation fortunately had a salutary effect and, when it ended in 1966, there had been a decided increase in the number vaccinated in all the areas under study.

That there should have been some waning of enthusiasm for BCG among the developed nations, with their highly organized health services and their declining incidence of tuberculosis, was understandable and logical. Indeed its incidence may ultimately reach a level at which continuance of community vaccination becomes unprofitable, a situation which was envisaged by Springett, a clinician with much statistical expertise and a member of the Medical Research Council's Vaccine Clinical Trials Committee, who said in his presidential address to the British Thoracic and Tuberculosis Association in 1971

I am quite seriously suggesting that a time is coming when BCG will be doing very little towards tuberculosis control in this country, and that

---

29 Guld, J. (1974) Some of the BCG trials and certain aspects involved in them. Correspondence. *Am. Rev. resp. Dis. 110*, 686.
30 Narain, R. (1974) *Ibid. 110*, 687.
31 Lotte, A., Perdrizet, S. & Hatton, F. (1971) Epidemiologie de la tuberculose et défaillances de la lutte anti-tuberculeuse chez l'enfant. *Bull. Wld Hlth Org. 44*, Supplement.

this will almost certainly be within the next 20 years. It may be closer in time than we realise . . .[32]

The question of the extent of the contribution which BCG can make to the tuberculosis problems of developing countries in Asia and Africa is still uncertain. Theoretically the contribution should be considerable and Crofton and Douglas two British authorities whose opinions command much respect do not hesitate to say: 'In economically developing countries BCG is probably one of the cheapest and most effective methods of tuberculosis control'.[33] Difficulties have been encountered, some of which have been attributable to deficiencies in the potency of the vaccine on exposure to tropical temperatures, but these have been largely eliminated by the substitution of the much more durable freeze-dried vaccine for the original short-lived liquid preparation. There is still uncertainty surrounding the degree of efficacy to be expected among communities where there is much low-grade tuberculin sensitivity and probable atypical mycobacterial infection, a situation which obtains in many tropical countries, but Hart considers that on present information it is reasonable to accept that BCG will have a moderate efficacy in the developing countries and 'that where there is a high tuberculosis risk a mass vaccination policy will make a worthwhile reduction in morbidity in the community.'[34]

Thus in over 50 years of experiment and experience the value of BCG has been established beyond doubt and, while there may be one or two questions which still lack a complete answer, hopes are justifiably high that there are benefits yet to come from the vaccine in the developing areas of the Third World. Although Albert Calmette died before the outstanding contribution which he made to the anti-tuberculosis campaign was internationally recognized his co-worker and constant collaborator, Camille Guérin, survived for a further 25 years to see the fruit of their original fortuitous observation yield an abundant harvest and to enjoy the acclaim and the honour which he shares with his distinguished colleague.

32 Springett, V. H. (1971) Tuberculosis control in Britain 1945–1970–1985 *Tubercle* *52*, 136.
33 Crofton, J. & Douglas, A. C. (1969) *Respiratory Diseases*. p. 187 London & Edinburgh: Blackwell.
34 Hart, P. D'A. (1967) Efficacy & applicability of mass BCG vaccination in tuberculosis control. *Br. med. J. 1*, 587.

Chapter Seventeen
Chemotherapy 1900-1945

In 1945, on the very eve of the greatest breakthrough in the history of tuberculosis, that distinguished American clinician, Max Pinner, wrote that

> there is no 'specific' treatment for tuberculosis, neither chemotherapeutic nor biological. During the last sixty years, innumerable compounds —many prepared according to planned therapeutic principles, many entirely empirical—have had their trials in animal experiments and in clinical work. Practically every chemical that has ever shown the slightest promise of benefit in any other infectious disease, has been tried in tuberculosis. Most metals in some chemical compound or other have been studied.[1]

This frenzy of therapeutic endeavour was a logical outcome to Koch's discovery of the bacillus while the subsequent failure of tuberculin to stimulate resistance to the disease at least stimulated science to even greater effort. Unfortunately most of the work was of the 'hit or miss' variety and was not marked by any very serious attempt at systematic research.

> Here and there in Europe were appearing reports of scanty experimental and uncontrolled clinical studies of various special preparations, especially of silica, calcium and guaiacol, each bearing some trade name and accredited with marvellous potencies which were not explained by the known properties of the components.[2]

Thus, in 1932, H. Gideon Wells summed up the early studies carried on outside the United States before recording the more scientific approach adopted by his colleague, Lydia De Witt, who explored the possibilities of iodides, chemotherapeutic dye compounds, guaiacol and

1 Pinner, M. (1945) *Pulmonary Tuberculosis in the Adult*. p. 424. Springfield, Ill: C. C. Thomas.
2 Wells, H. G. (1932) The chemotherapy of tuberculosis. *Yale J. Biol. Med.* 2, 611.

creosote, copper (including a most unwholesome sounding Japanese specific for tuberculosis which contained, amongst its other ingredients, two parts of potassium cyanide and one part of copper cyanurate) and various mercurial compounds. In none of these could she discern any gleam of hope for the future. Of all the minerals and metals studied during this period there were only two which may be said to have aroused widespread and sustained interest—calcium and gold.

The association of calcification with healed lesions and its absence in unhealed foci had been noted and recorded by the morbid anatomists, a point which was eventually seized upon by the clinicians, clutching desperately at any possible straw in their constantly losing battle with the disease. The first clinical observation bearing directly on the subject appears to have been that of Rénon when in 1906 he reported that in the village of Yonne, a limestone area where there had been lime-burning furnaces for ten years, no case of tuberculosis had been discovered amongst the 200 men employed in the industry in spite of the fact that the majority were alcholics.[3] Similar comment on the apparent excellent health and relative freedom from tuberculosis enjoyed by workers in the lime kilns in the vicinity of Edinburgh was made by Selkirk in 1908. He had been so impressed by his finding that he coupled with it the suggestion that such an occupation might be recommended 'to the working man predisposed to tuberculosis or already in the early stages of it', while he felt also that consideration might be given to the organization of a limeworks as a curative tuberculosis colony.[4] On the same theme Fisac, a Spanish physician, asserted in 1909 that 'all workers in lime and plaster of Paris are immune to tuberculosis in spite of the fact that they live in squalid dwellings and are underfed'.[5] Tweddell, intrigued by these comments from various sources in different countries, decided to pursue the matter further by writing to all the manufacturers of lime and plaster of Paris in the north-eastern United States, enquiring about the incidence of pulmonary tuberculosis among their employees. His enquiry met with a good response, many of the replies coming from physicians employed by the companies, and all to the effect that

3   Renon, L. (1906) *Bull. méd., Paris. 20*, 924. (Quoted by Brockbank, W. (1926–27) Observations on the serum calcium in pulmonary tuberculosis. *Q. J. Med. 20*, 431.)
4   Selkirk, W. J. B. (1908) Tuberculosis in limeworkers. *Br. med. J. 2*, 1493.
5   Fisac (1900) Quoted by Tweddell, F. (1922) The need of calcium-therapy in tuberculosis. *Med. Rec.* 141.

tuberculosis was unknown amongst their work-force. This information led Tweddell to postulate the existence of an immunity to tuberculosis resulting from the continual inhalation of finely divided particles of lime and gypsum.

> Lime in contact with water or the moist tissues of the lungs forms calcium hydroxide, which acts as a caustic and antiseptic and is then absorbed ... This action appears to be specific in early pulmonary tuberculosis, for some unknown reason, the same as quinine is specific for malaria.[6]

A more critical and scientific study was that conducted by Miriam Iszard who, after an exhaustive survey of the literature, concluded that

> the statistical data of the United States show that tuberculosis mortality is higher for all calcium dust industries than for the population as a whole. The percentage, however, is markedly lower than for those industries involving exposure to dust of high silica content.

After a series of experiments in which rabbits exposed to calcium hydrate dust were subsequently infected with tubercle bacilli she reported that the pulmonary lesions which followed had developed slightly more slowly than in the controls but were otherwise indistinguishable.[7] This finding could hardly have been termed encouraging but the clinicians, if they had little else, had unbounded faith and so their patients received calcium.

Given at first by mouth until it was realized that its absorption from the alimentary tract was so poor as to make oral administration quite useless, calcium was later given mainly by intravenous injection—a much more impressive performance which no doubt made a major contribution to its efficacy. Calcium therapy attained much popularity in continental clinics where its use continued long after all doubts as to its value had been resolved. It was never employed on such a lavish scale in Britain although Brockbank, working at the Brompton Hospital, felt that it had something to offer[8] and Prest, the medical superintendent of a Scottish sanatorium, wrote about it with an enthusiasm which was as unrestrained as it was uncritical.[9] The position

6 Tweddell, F. (5).
7 Iszard, M. S. (1925) Calcium and tuberculosis. *J. ind. Hyg. 7*, 505.
8 Brockbank, W. (1926–27) Observations on the serum calcium in pulmonary tuberculosis and on treatment by intravenous injections of calcium. *Q. J. Med. 20*, 431.
9 Prest, E. E. (1922) The treatment of tuberculosis with colloid of calcium. *Lancet 1*, 53.

which calcium finally came to occupy in the treatment of tuberculosis was well summarized by Maurice Davidson, physician to the Brompton Hospital, when he wrote in 1935:

> In common with others we have seen cases in which reduction of the temperature has occurred, together with a certain amount of improvement in the general condition of phthisical patients, after a long spell of calcium therapy, and it can at least be said that the treatment, which is perfectly harmless, is worth a trial in cases in which the practitioner is hard put to it to respond to the insistent demand that something further should be done for the bed-ridden patient.[10]

While calcium was, for practical purposes, an inert medicament which neither benefited nor harmed the patient, the gold salts which were introduced into treatment in the early 1920s posed a very different problem. Gold therapy was not a new idea but merely the resurrection of an old one for since ancient days gold had been used at one time or another as a treatment for practically every known disease, including tuberculosis—a tribute more to its precious character and regal status than to any proven curative properties. De Witt and her associates investigated the therapeutic value of various gold salts in experimental tuberculosis in guinea-pigs, including a gold canthariden compound introduced for clinical use in Germany by Speiss and Feldt between 1912 and 1916, but found none which had any notable effect on the disease except that life in general was shorter and the disease more pronounced in the treated animals than in the controls.[11]

Whether this careful work was known to or simply ignored by Holger Møllgaard of Copenhagen when, in 1924, he introduced sanocrysin, is not clear. He had for some time been investigating the therapeutic usefulness of a variety of heavy metals and in the course of this study he produced an inorganic compound, a double thiosulphate of gold and sodium, which he named sanocrysin and which he claimed had a specific and frequently beneficial action on tuberculous disease. He did not suggest that either the specificity or the benefit resulted from any direct bactericidal action of the gold salt but held that events were influenced favourably through the medium

---

10 Davidson, M. (1935) *A Practical Manual of Diseases of the Chest.* p. 362. London: Oxford University Press.
11 Wells, H. G. (2).

of the violent reaction which sanocrysin injection provoked. In his own words:

> It is a well-known fact that the injection of sanocrysin into an animal infected with tuberculosis causes a violent reaction which appears clinically as acute intoxication of the organism. The symptoms are albuminuria, myocarditis and fall in temperature. In other cases there is no shock but high temperature reactions. I regarded both these reactions as reactions of immunity, due to liberation of toxins from dissolved tubercle bacilli and from tuberculous tissue, and I suggested that the shock is the reaction of the non-immune organism and the rise in temperature the reaction of the partially immune organism to these toxins. The foundation for this interpretation is the fact that the shock can be removed by the intravenous injection of a specific tuberculosis serum made by immunizing cattle with tubercle bacilli, and that it is possible by prophylactic injection of this serum to remove a tuberculous animal from a state in which shock is to be expected to the condition in which it responds to sanocrysin with a rise of temperature.[12]

However ominous Møllgaard's theories may have sounded his work attracted attention and when encouraging results were reported by Knud Secher, the first to use sanocrysin in clinical practice, the attention was transformed into interest and even a modest degree of excitement. The fact that Secher was a general physician working in a general hospital, whose tuberculous patients were mainly observation cases destined for transfer to a sanatorium, failed to lessen the impact of his pronouncements.

Hard on Secher's heels came Knud Faber, professor of clinical medicine in the University of Copenhagen, who began to use sanocrysin in the university clinic at the beginning of 1925. Employing a dosage schedule which was later recognized to be far too high he recorded some hair-raising episodes.

> We were prepared to see serious consequences follow the sanocrysin injections in severe cases in view of the already published experiences. In the first few weeks we also had cases in which the reactions caused by the treatment could not be controlled, so that the patient succumbed before he otherwise would have done.[13]

Faber was convinced that he had succeeded in overcoming the main difficulties but his account of those reactions which he came to regard

12 Møllgaard, H. (1926–27) Some of the principal questions in chemotherapy with special regard to heavy metals. *Proc. R. Soc. Med. 20*, 787.
13 Faber, K. (1925) Treatment of phthisis with sanocrysin. *Lancet 2*, 62.

as inseparable from the therapy, painted a frightening picture of the tribulations which must have been endured by his patients. High fever, anorexia, nausea, vomiting, albuminuria, skin eruptions and polyarthralgia were all accepted by him as a reasonable price to pay for results which he described thus: 'In a certain number of patients the favourable effect was very striking, in others it was more doubtful, and in some it could not be detected'.

Other Danish physicians appear to have learnt rapidly that sano-crysin must be approached with caution. Würtzen and Permin, both of whom had at the beginning employed it extensively, lost their enthusiasm and Permin, who came to favour small doses at regular intervals, is quoted by Kayne as saying that, in view of the possible benefit to be derived, he 'did not feel justified in withholding it.'[14] In most Norwegian and Swedish centres, after traumatic experiences with the dosage recommended by Secher and Faber, sanocrysin plummeted from favour and was virtually discarded but protagonists emerged elsewhere in Europe, notably Sayé in Barcelona and Leon Bernard at the Laënnec Hospital in Paris. The decade 1925–35 saw the period of the 'gold rush' for sanocrysin caught the public imagina-tion; most tuberculosis physicians made some use of it and a volu-minous literature was built up, reaching a peak in 1934–35. A decline in the volume of published work then set in, a decline which accelerated rapidly and which may well have been influenced by the fact that in 1934–35 fully one-third of the papers appearing dealt primarily with the toxic effects of the treatment.[15]

In none of the early European work had any attempt been made to carry out a controlled trial of sanocrysin, an important omission which was later to be rectified by American workers when, in 1931, Amber-son, McMahon and Pinner published the results of a clinical trial which had been strictly controlled. They found no convincing evi-dence that sanocrysin conferred any notable benefit on its recipients and laid considerable stress on the high incidence of associated toxic complications.[16] The succeeding years produced no further enlighten-ment and Goldberg, in his authoritative textbook, was impelled to write that he felt unable to recommend 'the use of this substance and

14 Kayne, G. G. (1936) The use of sanocrysin in the treatment of pulmonary tuberculosis. *Proc. R. Soc. Med. 28*, 1463.

15 Hart, P. D'A. (1946) Chemotherapy of tuberculosis. *Br. med. J. 2*, 805.

16 Amberson, J. B., McMahon, B. T. & Pinner, M. (1931) A clinical trial of sanocrysin in pulmonary tuberculosis. *Am. Rev. Tuberc. 24*, 401.

other similar compounds until more adequate data concerning its utilization can be established in preventing the serious complications that we have met.'[17]

In Britain the majority of tuberculosis physicians acquired some experience of sanocrysin but there was no evidence of any wild enthusiasm over the results. A typical publication of the period came in 1932 from Mansell, working at the Brompton Hospital, who reported on a series of 153 patients treated between 1926 and 1928 and concluded that 'in cases of extensive exudative disease sanocrysin in small doses often has a beneficial immediate effect which may be at least of economic value. There is yet no convincing evidence that this effect is lasting . . .'[18]

By 1939 the position was substantially unchanged. The exact mode of action of sanocrysin remained unknown, the dosage was in dispute and there was no firm agreement on the indications for its employment. There were, indeed, experienced physicians who doubted whether it should ever be used at all and it was quite clear that the gold fever had spent itself. By 1943 sanocrysin, as far as the treatment of tuberculosis was concerned, was well on the way to oblivion.

In a retrospective survey in 1946 D'Arcy Hart commented: 'This astonishing acceptance of a remedy and its subsequent rejection without any immediate better substitute, is only equalled by the preceding . . . dramatic rise and fall of tuberculin therapy.' Among the possible explanations for this precipitate slump in gold therapy he has suggested the following:

(1) The laboratory groundwork on the curative effect of sanocrysin was insecure, and the drug was heavily sponsored for general therapeutic use without adequately critical clinical trials. (2) The drug's toxicity relative to presumed effective dose was at first underrated. (3) The clinical benefit was not dramatic or constant enough to dispense with balanced controls, which were in fact rarely used, and where they were . . . the results were discouraging.[19]

While gold was glissading down from its 1935 peak interest in the discovery of a chemotherapeutic solution to the problem of tuberculosis was being kept alive by the latest work on the sulphonamides.

17   Goldberg, B. (1939) *Clinical Tuberculosis* C–76. Philadelphia: F. A. Davis.
18   Mansell, H. E. (1932) On the use of sanocrysin in pulmonary tuberculosis. *Lancet*. 2, 837.
19   Hart, P. D'A. (15).

Although much had already been accomplished in protozoal and spirochaetal infections, the action of the sulphonamides signalled the first major breach in the *bacterial* front. The efficacy of these new sulpha drugs in acute infections, their diffusibility and the presumption that their point of attack was the bacteria themselves, led naturally and rapidly to the investigation of their potentialities against the tubercle bacillus. The first to be tested was sulphanilamide which was found by Rich and Follis, when administered in large doses, to have an inhibitory effect on tuberculosis in experimental animals.[20] Unfortunately neither sulphanilamide nor others of the sulphonamide series showed any real promise when tested in the clinical field.[21] A brief gleam of hope followed the introduction of the more complex sulphone compounds, and promin in particular gave very encouraging results in Feldman's laboratory at the Mayo Clinic[22] and in Medlar's at Bellevue Hospital[23] but these experimental results were, unfortunately, not borne out in clinical practice.[24]

Further studies of the sulphone group had been planned and were proceeding when the whole direction of the attack was switched following the demonstration of the almost ideal chemotherapeutic properties of penicillin. No other antibiotic substance had as yet proved of undoubted efficacy in clinical medicine but, with the unveiling of penicillin, the floodgates of research into this branch of microbiology were thrown wide open and it soon became clear that it was only a matter of time before someone somewhere would discover an antibiotic capable of dealing with tuberculosis as penicillin was dealing with acute bacterial infections.

20 Rich, A. R. & Follis, R. H. (1938) The inhibitory effect of sulfanilamide on the development of experimental tuberculosis in the guinea-pig. *Bull. Johns Hopkins Hosp.* *62*, 77.

21 Zucker, G., Pinner, M. & Hyman, H. T. (1942) Chemotherapy of tuberculosis. *Am. Rev. Tuberc. 45*, 292; *46*, 277.

22 Feldman, W. H. (1942) Promin in experimental tuberculosis. *Am. Rev. Tuberc. 45*, 303; *46*, 187.

23 Medlar, E. M. & Sasano, K. T. (1943) Promin in experimental tuberculosis in the guinea-pig. *Am. Rev. Tuberc. 47*, 618.

24 Hinshaw, H. C., Pfuetze, K. & Feldman, W. H. (1943) Treatment of tuberculosis with promin. *Am. Rev. Tuberc. 47*, 26.

Chapter Eighteen
The Rainbow's End: Streptomycin, P.A.S. and Isoniazid

The signal honour of discovering an antibiotic effective against *Mycobacterium tuberculosis* fell, not to a physician who happened also to be a scientist, but to a non-medical professor of microbiology—an indication of the increasing complexity and wide ramifications of research programmes directed towards the production of new antibacterial agents.

Selman Abraham Waksman was born in the Ukraine in 1888. He received his early education at Odessa and later, after emigrating to the United States in 1910, attended Rutgers University where he graduated with the degree of M.Sc. in 1916, becoming a naturalized American citizen in that same year. After a period of postgraduate study leading to a Ph.D. in biochemistry from the University of California he returned to his old university as lecturer in soil microbiology. In 1925 he became associate professor of microbiology and, continuing on the upward path, was appointed full professor and head of the department in 1930, serving in this post and as director of the Institute of Microbiology until his retirement in 1958.

After the deaths of Alexander Fleming and Howard Florey, Waksman became and remained the outstanding world figure among the pioneers of antibiotic discovery. Having been for a long time interested in the study of intermicrobial antagonism he isolated and purified two antibiotics, actinomycin in 1940 and streptothricin in 1942, although both, unfortunately, proved too toxic to be of therapeutic value. But his greatest triumph was not to be long delayed and January 1944 found him writing that 'A new antibacterial substance, designated as streptomycin, was isolated from two strains of an actinomyces related to an organism described as *Actinomyces griseus*'.[1]

1 Schatz, A., Bugie, B. & Waksman, S. A. (1944) Streptomycin, a substance exhibiting antibiotic activity against Gram-positive and Gram-negative bacteria. *Proc. Soc. exp. Biol. Med. 55*, 66.

The remainder of that year was devoted to detailed exploration of the field of action of his latest antibiotic and in November came the first disclosure of its *in vitro* bacteriostatic action against *M. tuberculosis*.[2] Before making this announcement Waksman had already enlisted the aid of two colleagues who were to be responsible for the next phase of the exploration—that of animal experiment and of clinical trial— and events were to demonstrate the wisdom of his choice. The rapidity and scientific accuracy with which these investigations were planned and executed reflected the greatest credit upon the scientist and the physician responsible and brought fresh renown to the world-famous institution in which they both worked.

The animal experiments were under the control of William Hugh Feldman, professor of comparative pathology in the Mayo Foundation, who had already formulated, during his work on the sulphone group, the principles which should guide any investigator attempting the laboratory evaluation of an antituberculosis drug. Born in Glasgow in 1892 as William Hugh Gunn he emigrated with his family to the United States in 1894 and, after his father's death and mother's re-marriage, took the name of his stepfather. He obtained his D.V.M. degree at the Colorado State College in 1917 and his M.Sc. followed nine years later. In 1927 he was appointed professor of comparative pathology in the Mayo Foundation and became head of the department of experimental pathology in the Foundation's Institute of Experimental Medicine in 1947. His clinical colleague was Horton Corwin Hinshaw. Originally a bacteriologist with the degree of Ph.D. from the University of California, Hinshaw obtained his M.D. from the University of Pennsylvania in 1933 and thereafter, devoting his attention to clinical medicine, became a consultant physician at the Mayo Clinic and associate professor of medicine in the Mayo Foundation. Together Feldman and Hinshaw formed a powerful and authoritative team and before the end of 1944 they had produced the next link in the chain of evidence with a joint paper describing the *in vivo* suppressive effect of streptomycin on the development and course of tuberculous disease in laboratory animals. After describing their experiments they considered that the results justified the conclusion

that streptomycin is an antibiotic substance which is well tolerated by

2 Schatz, A. & Waksman, S. A. (1944) Effect of streptomycin and other antibiotic substances upon mycobacterium tuberculosis and related organisms. *Proc. Soc. exp. Biol. Med.* *57*, 244.

guinea pigs and which, under the conditions imposed, exerts a striking suppressive effect on the pathogenic proclivities of the human variety of *M. tuberculosis* in guinea pigs.[3]

Thus, within 12 months of the announcement of its isolation, the antituberculosis action of streptomycin had been clearly and unequivocally demonstrated both *in vitro* and *in vivo*.

The admirable restraint and caution shown by those concerned in this crucial research project indicated how well the lessons of the past had been learnt. No premature publicity such as that which had surrounded Koch and his tuberculin was permitted, while the basic laboratory experimentation, so sketchily performed in the case of sanocrysin, was planned and executed with a care which invested the findings with complete authority. Fortified with such laboratory evidence there was clearly no need to delay the search for the ultimate proof which only a clinical trial could provide.

The amount of streptomycin which Waksman could produce was small and this consideration, added to the fact that knowledge of its pharmacological properties was incomplete, called for great caution and a very restricted dosage was employed initially. No definite evidence of benefit was detectable but, with the aid of information provided by a concomitant study of the pharmacology,[4] clearer guides for its therapeutic use emerged. Thereafter an increase in dose produced more encouraging results and, in September 1945, Hinshaw and Feldman issued a guarded preliminary report to the effect that from a study of 34 patients who had tuberculosis and who had received streptomycin

> it appears probable that streptomycin has exerted a limited suppressive effect, especially on some of the more unusual types of pulmonary and extrapulmonary tuberculosis in this small series of patients. While the reproduction of *M. tuberculosis* may have been temporarily inhibited by the treatment administered, we obtained no convincing evidence of rapidly effective bactericidal action.

This historic communication on the use of streptomycin in clinical tuberculosis ended with a plea which was indicative of the great responsibility felt by the writers:

3 Feldman, W. H. & Hinshaw, H. C. (1944) Effects of streptomycin on experimental tuberculosis in guinea-pigs: A preliminary report. *Proc. Staff Meet. Mayo Clin. 19*, 593.
4 Heilman, D. H. et al. (1945) Streptomycin: absorption, diffusion, excretion and toxicity. *Am. J. med. Sci. 210*, 576.

It is to be ardently hoped that if these results are noticed by lay persons, they will interpret the results in the same cautious frame of mind that the scientific investigators have endeavoured to maintain. This unusual suggestion is made for the benefit of the many thousands of patients who have tuberculosis. Morale plays a crucial part in treatment of such a debilitating and chronic disease, and morale is injured by premature and optimistic reports of results which may not be sustained in practice. No one as yet knows what the final judgment will be concerning the effect of streptomycin on clinical tuberculosis.[5]

Apart from the fact that this report came from two workers already held in high esteem by their colleagues the very caution with which its tentative conclusions were presented added to its authority and aroused world-wide interest. The work of the Mayo Clinic group continued and by the early part of 1946 it was clear that streptomycin held much promise and that extensive clinical tests were now not only justified but indicated. There was no lack of organizations or individuals willing and anxious to undertake such trials but the fact that streptomycin was both scarce and expensive imposed a useful curb on an enthusiasm which could have become as misdirected as it was uninhibited.

The major pharmaceutical manufacturers had naturally been interested in the new antibiotic from an early stage and, with their technical expertise, had quickly succeeded in producing a purer and less toxic preparation than that originally supplied to the Mayo Foundation by Waksman: by the autumn of 1946 sufficient had been manufactured to permit an expansion of clinical and laboratory research. The twin factors of scarcity and high cost pointed to the need for some form of control over the distribution of the supplies available, a task undertaken by a federal organization, the Civilian Production Administration. With the blessing of this organization six of the leading manufacturers of streptomycin approached the American Trudeau Society (the clinical off-shoot of the National Tuberculosis Association) and offered to provide a supply of the antibiotic if the Society would arrange a programme of research and clinical trials. This offer was accepted with alacrity and plans for the proposed trials were drawn up for submission to the Society's Committee on Medical Research which, in October 1946, gave the project its full support. Throughout the course of this Trudeau Society

5 Hinshaw, H. C. & Feldman, W. H. (1945) Streptomycin in treatment of clinical tuberculosis: a preliminary report. *Proc. Staff. Meet. Mayo Clin.* 20, 313.

investigation more than a million dollars worth of streptomycin was donated to the Society by the Streptomycin Producers Association.[6]

Another project which was developing throughout 1946 had been initiated in June of that year by the federal agencies most closely concerned with the treatment of tuberculosis, the Veterans Administration, the Army and the Navy, which, acting through a Joint Streptomycin Committee for Tuberculosis, co-operated in what was to develop into one of the most extensive research studies ever mounted. The importance of correlating the work of the federal agencies with that of the Trudeau Society was fully appreciated by both parties and satisfactory liaison for the exchange of information and ideas was established, not only with each other but also with the Mayo Clinic group and with a smaller study, directed primarily at the toxicity of streptomycin, which was proceeding at Cornell University Medical College under the guidance of Walsh McDermott.[7]

With the launching of these activities a steady flow of information was generated and in August 1947 McLeod Riggins, the reigning president of the Trudeau Society, and Corwin Hinshaw, in reviewing the progress which had been made, considered that there was sufficient sound evidence to warrant the following conclusions:

(1) Streptomycin exerts unprecedented therapeutic effects upon well-established experimental tuberculosis in guinea-pigs. Under some conditions it is possible to eradicate the disease in a considerable proportion of animals, even though the disease has been permitted to develop to an advanced stage prior to institution of treatment.

(2) Streptomycin is the first antibacterial drug which has shown definitely promising results in the treatment of certain types of pulmonary and extrapulmonary tuberculosis in man.

(3) Under certain circumstances streptomycin appears to lessen or to prevent further multiplication of tubercle bacilli in lesions of human tuberculosis, but usually this suppressive effect is of limited duration. After a few weeks or months of continuous treatment streptomycin-resistant tubercle bacilli may appear and fail to yield to streptomycin therapy. Fortunately, there are types of tuberculosis in which only temporary suppression of the infection is necessary in order to permit natural defensive mechanisms to gain ascendency . . .

(4) During its period of effective action, streptomycin administration

6 National Tuberculosis Association (1959) Tuberculosis Medical Research 1904–1955. N.Y. Nat. Tuberc. Ass. p. 66.
7 Report to the Council on Pharmacy & Chemistry (1947) The effects of streptomycin on tuberculosis in man. *J. Am. med. Ass. 135*, 634.

frequently results in marked amelioration of symptoms of pulmonary tuberculosis . . .

(5) In the highly fatal types of generalized tuberculosis including miliary tuberculosis and tuberculous meningitis, streptomycin frequently brings about a striking clinical, roentgenographic and bacteriological remission. Unfortunately, this state of remission may continue for only a few months, but a small number of patients with otherwise fatal tuberculous meningitis have remained well for more than a year without evidence of recurrence of their disease. It is now widely believed that treatment with streptomycin is mandatory in early cases of miliary tuberculosis and tuberculous meningitis . . .

(6) Marked improvement has frequently been noted in previously progressive cases of ulcerating tuberculosis involving the larynx, the trachea and the larger bronchi.

(7) Chronic, long-standing tuberculous lesions involving lymph nodes, the thoracic wall, et cetera, with sinus tracts which have drained pus for months or years, frequently subside within a few weeks following streptomycin treatment. Some of these may recur.

(11) The toxic reaction most frequently encountered is a disturbance of equilibrium, which is uncomfortable but usually not dangerous. In most instances it has been extremely mild, and in a few it has been severe. In all instances, a satisfactory degree of recovery or compensation to this condition has occurred. . . . Deafness has been known to occur, but nearly all such instances have been in patients with tuberculous meningitis and probably would not have occurred but for the necessity of continued treatment in high dosage without interruption, due to the otherwise fatal nature of the disease . . .

(13) A great deal remains to be learned about the ways in which streptomycin may be employed more effectively. The optimum dosage schedules have not yet been determined, and the maximum duration of treatment is not definitely known. There is considerable evidence to suggest that often marked symptomatic and definite roentgenographic and bacteriological improvement may follow the administration of smaller doses of streptomycin than generally used heretofore. One or two grams daily, given for periods of 42 to 120 days, depending in part on whether or not the organisms become drug resistant, may bring about remission of the disease . . .[8]

This appreciation of the situation, while conveying much encouragement also illuminated clearly the problems which had yet to be solved before streptomycin could be hailed as the miracle for

8 Riggins, H. M. & Hinshaw, H. C. (1947) The streptomycin–tuberculosis research project of the American Trudeau Society. *Am. Rev. Tuberc. 96*, 168.

which the world had been waiting. In November 1947 the federal
agencies also issued a preliminary report which was couched in somewhat similar terms—encouraging but cautious over toxicity and
gravely concerned about the apparent inevitability with which
resistance to the drug developed with consequent disintegration of
its therapeutic usefulness.

This concern was all the more acute since little was known about
the genesis of resistance.

> There is some evidence that it is due to the survival and multiplication of
> a small number of inherently resistant organisms rather than being an
> acquired phenomenon. If this is the case the discovery of another drug to
> which these few organisms are sensitive would appear necessary to
> overcome the phenomenon.[9]

Thus two planned and co-ordinated investigations had at this early
stage brought to light one of the major problems associated with
streptomycin treatment, a problem which was to prove probably the
greatest of all those associated with the chemotherapy of tuberculosis
and which could only be solved by the exercise of the most unremit-
ting care and attention in each individual case.

Since the discovery of streptomycin had been an American achievement it was but natural and just that the country of its origin should
have enjoyed priority in the exciting adventure which the early
exploration of its possibilities involved. The preliminary reports in the
American journals ignited world-wide interest while Europe, grappling with a massive tuberculosis problem, wondered if salvation
might be at hand. In Britain concern about the war-time increase in
tuberculosis was compounded by the anxiety and embarrassment
associated with the national post-war impoverishment, a financial
constraint which made it imperative that any precious dollars
allocated for the purchase of streptomycin be expended to the best
advantage. The Medical Research Council had been allotted a small
supply of the antibiotic and, mindful of past history, made its decision.
No one knew better than the members of the Council that the natural
course of pulmonary tuberculosis 'is in fact so variable and unpredictable that evidence of improvement or cure following the use of a new
drug in a few cases cannot be accepted as proof of the effect of that
drug'[10] and they cited the exaggerated claims which had been made

9 Report to the Council on Pharmacy & Chemistry (7).
10 Medical Research Council Investigation (1948) Streptomycin treatment of pulmonary
tuberculosis. *Br. med. J.* 2, 1073.

for gold therapy over so many years as a spectacular example of such self-deception. They had noted with some surprise that the elaborate American investigations which were proceeding did not include a controlled trial and they decided that the British allocation could be most profitably expended on a rigorously planned investigation which included concurrent controls. An expert committee, the Streptomycin Trials Committee, was set up to plan and supervize this work. The trial started in January 1947 and was meticulously planned, organized and executed. It set patterns and standards for subsequent trials, both in the United Kingdom and overseas, and may fairly be regarded as marking a turning point in the scientific assessment of drugs alleged to possess curative properties in tuberculous disease.

The Committee issued its first report in October 1948, a report which provided the clearest possible proof that the course of bilateral acute progressive tuberculosis could be halted by streptomycin treatment. Fifty-one per cent of the streptomycin-treated patients had shown considerable radiological improvement: that streptomycin was the factor responsible for this improvement was attested by the results in the control group wherein only 8 per cent had shown a similar favourable change. The major improvement had occurred during the first two to three months of treatment; in the latter half of the period of observation, which extended to six months, many of the participants showed evidence of deterioration, a finding which was believed to be linked with the emergence of streptomycin resistant strains among the infecting organisms. The Committee drew the conclusion that 'it seems fair to assume that after two to three months of streptomycin treatment in a patient with open pulmonary tuberculosis further treatment or a repeat course later is unlikely to be effective' and that 'organized investigation will be needed to determine whether emergence of streptomycin-resistant strains can be prevented by association of streptomycin with another drug or by a special rhythm of treatment'.

By the latter part of 1948, only four and a half years after Waksman's original announcement of his discovery, American and British research workers had produced incontrovertible evidence of the specific antibacterial action of streptomycin on *M. tuberculosis* but they had also dispelled any hopes of an easy and painless victory by delineating streptomycin's limitations and hazards. All were agreed that it must be employed without hesitation in those hitherto fatal forms of tuberculosis, meningitis and miliary disease, in which it could be life-saving. In the management of patients with the more acute type of pulmonary disease it was seen mainly as a means of converting them into acceptable risks for collapse therapy which involved giving streptomycin for a few weeks only, stopping short of the point at which resistance might be expected to develop. It appeared to have little to offer the patient with chronic pulmonary tuberculosis—that extensive field in which help was most urgently required.

Both the British Medical Research Council's report and that of the federal agencies in the United States had embodied some speculative thoughts on the possibility of overcoming the problem of streptomycin resistance by the discovery of another drug to which the resistant bacilli were sensitive and which might be incorporated with streptomycin in the treatment regimen. The opportunity to put this theory to the proof was not to be longed delayed.

Jorgen Lehmann, working at the Sahlgrenska Hospital in Gothenburg, had been engaged in following up earlier studies by Bernheim who had shown that oxygen uptake by pathogenic strains of *M. tuberculosis* was stimulated both by benzoic and salicylic acids. Lehmann now embarked on a search for competitive inhibitors of these acids and eventually established that *para*-aminosalicylic acid had demonstrable bacteriostatic activity *in vitro* against *M. tuberculosis*. Animal experiments were begun and also a small clinical trial which, starting in March 1944, involved 20 patients. In a preliminary communication in January 1946 Lehmann reported that the majority of the patients had responded favourably with a decrease in temperature and in the erythrocyte sedimentation rate accompanying an improvement in their general condition.[11]

The general awareness that streptomycin resistance constituted a major and unsolved problem meant that much attention was focussed on Lehmann's report and a number of small, unofficial and uncontrolled trials were begun. In Britain these produced conflicting results and, mindful of the decisive answer reached in the streptomycin trial, the Ministry of Health and the British Tuberculosis Association approached the Medical Research Council with the request that *para*-aminosalicylic acid (P.A.S.) should be submitted to a like process of investigation. The Council agreed to this request and again remitted the detailed planning to their Streptomycin Trials Committee on which some members of the Tuberculosis Association's

11 Lehmann, J. (1946) *Para*-aminosalicylic acid in the treatment of tuberculosis. *Lancet 1*, 15.

Research Committee were invited to serve. On this occasion it was clear that, in view of the proven efficacy of streptomycin in the forms of tuberculosis most suitable for chemotherapy trials, an investigation which employed for comparison a control group treated by bed-rest only would no longer be possible. The Committee resolved instead 'to compare the effect of P.A.S. treatment in one group of patients with the effect of streptomycin in another group having similar disease'. Further as it seemed possible that the combination of P.A.S. with streptomycin might delay or prevent the emergence of strepto-mycin resistance it was decided to have three concurrent groups, the treatment being in the first group P.A.S. alone, in the second group streptomycin alone, and in the third a combination of the two drugs. The does of P.A.S., given orally, was fixed at 5 g four times daily, and of streptomycin at 1 g daily, given as a single injection each morning. The chemotherapy was to continue for three months and was then to be followed by one month's observation, with the patient on bed-rest only, after which any other treatment might be initiated.

The trial began in December 1948 and the final report was issued in November 1950 but, as the work proceeded, information of such importance emerged that the Council felt obliged in the public interest to authorize a brief preliminary statement. Issued on 31 December 1949 this was to the effect that

> the trial has demonstrated unequivocally that the combination of P.A.S. with streptomycin reduces considerably the risk of development of streptomycin-resistant strains of tubercle bacilli during the six months following the start of treatment. This conclusion is applicable so far only to the acute forms of disease treated, and it remains to be seen whether the same results are obtainable in other forms of the disease amenable to streptomycin therapy. Furthermore, the conclusion is applicable only to the large doses of P.A.S. used; this dosage causes discomfort in some patients, and it has been agreed to find out, by further trials, whether smaller doses would achieve the same result.[12]

No retraction of this preliminary observation was required when the full report was published 11 months later.

> 'It is now possible to adjudge the place of P.A.S. in the chemotherapy of pulmonary tuberculosis . . . P.A.S. given alone has a place in the treat-ment of cases which show apparently complete streptomycin resistance.

---

12 Medical Research Council Investigation (1949) Treatment of pulmonary tuberculosis with *para*-aminosalicylic acid and streptomycin: preliminary report. *Br. med. J.* 2, 1521.

The most important conclusion concerns the use of combined therapy. In view of its effect on streptomycin resistance, it is obvious that the addition of P.A.S. prolongs the period of effective streptomycin treatment . . . Combination of P.A.S. with streptomycin not only renders effective administration of streptomycin possible for longer periods than previously, but probably permits also of repeated effective courses. The use of chemotherapy thereby becomes justifiable for a wider range of lesions.'[13]

With the publication of this report the bogey of streptomycin resistance began to recede but the time when the new chemotherapy could be regarded as definitive treatment in its own right, other than for tuberculous meningitis and miliary tuberculosis, still seemed far distant. For the moment it was warmly welcomed by the thoracic surgeons as a means of expediting operations such as thoracoplasty.

Heretofore, in those cases which were unstable—cases during a relapse and the slipping chronics—only bed-rest was at our disposal in attempting to stabilize them; now, however, antibiotics had changed the position; cases which needed many months of preparation can now be so prepared in a matter of weeks.[14]

In addition to its value in the classical collapse therapy procedures, it gave a fresh impetus to the treatment of tuberculosis by lung resection.

The use of streptomycin is regarded as essential in patients undergoing resection of tuberculous lung, and while some of the improved results of these operations are due to better technique, it is generally accepted that streptomycin has played an important part in reducing the incidence of complications.[15]

While these were important entries on the credit side of the therapeutic ledger, honest accounting required that due weight be given also to those on the debit side, which were concerned chiefly with the toxic effects produced in a proportion of patients by both streptomycin and P.A.S. Those associated with streptomycin were already known but the unpleasant gastrointestinal symptoms produced by P.A.S. in the currently stipulated dose of 20 g daily placed a great

13   Medical Research Council Investigation (1950) Treatment of pulmonary tuberculosis with streptomycin and *para*-aminosalicylic acid. *Br. med. J.* 2, 1073.
14   Sellors, T. H. & Livingstone, J. L. (1952) *Modern Practice in Tuberculosis*. Vol. ii, p. 116. London: Butterworth.
15   *Ibid.* Vol. i, p. 311.

strain on the patient's fortitude and endurance while the liability of both products to initiate hypersensitivity reactions, some of considerable severity, was not yet fully apparent.

While the surgeons rejoiced in the greater freedom of action which they now enjoyed the physicians still longed wistfully for the day when some genius would produce another antituberculosis drug, one which would be effective, cheap, easily administered and at least relatively non-toxic—an ideal as entrancing as it seemed unattainable. In fact, though, the day when such a discovery was to be made lay just immediately ahead and it also marked the passing of an era when nearly all discoveries or advances (the terms are not necessarily synonymous) in the field of tuberculosis had resulted from the effort of a single individual, often working in relative isolation.

The complex nature and high cost of modern chemotherapeutic research was proving too much for the individual worker, usually relying on very modest grants from university or government sources, and he was being replaced by research teams maintained and equipped by the giant pharmaceutical companies who had so much to gain from success. In the period following the introduction of streptomycin and P.A.S. such organizations were humming with activity and the discovery of the next major antituberculosis agent is said to have been made more or less simultaneously by three groups of workers at Hoffman La Roche and at the Squibb Institute for Medical Research, both in the United States, and at the Farbenfabriken Bayer in Germany.[16]

An observation which had been made during the course of investigative work on the thiosemicarbazones had led, during 1950–51, to the testing for antituberculosis activity of isonicotinic acid hydrazide. So hopeful were the laboratory results that an initial clinical trial appeared to be fully justified and this was begun at Sea View Hospital, New York, in the latter half of 1951. In 1952 Robitzek and Selikoff assessed the response to this drug of 44 consecutive patients with 'acute active progressive bilateral caseous-pneumonic tuberculosis' all of whom were continuously febrile, were losing weight, had sputum which was constantly positive and in general were regarded as having an extremely poor prognosis. Under treatment with oral isonicotinic acid hydrazide all showed marked general improvement with a rapid fall in temperature, a significant gain in weight and an

16 Barry, V. C. (1964) *Chemotherapy of Tuberculosis.* p. 49. London: Butterworth.

increased sense of well-being. In addition cough and sputum diminished and the bacillary content of the latter decreased, while in a proportion of the patients X-ray examination showed a reduction in size of pre-treatment cavities. Such a response not unnaturally led Robitzek and Selikoff to the conclusion that isonicotinic acid hydrazide exerted 'an impressive effect upon the course of acute caseous-pneumonic tuberculosis in humans'.[17] No comparable control series had been included in this trial and, although resistance study results were not available at the time of publication, the authors claimed that no clinical evidence which might indicate the onset of resistance had been noted by them even in patients who had had more than three and a half months therapy.

Unlike streptomycin, isonicotinic acid hydrazide, soon to be more conveniently named isoniazid, had to endure the hardship of premature and unauthorized publicity. Even before publication of the preliminary report by Robitzek and Selikoff the unit at Sea View Hospital had been invaded by reporters who, having talked to patients, proceeded to hit the headlines, supporting the printed word by photographs of previously dying patients dancing in the wards after receiving a course of the new 'miracle drug'. The presentation lacked nothing in the way of sensationalism, irresponsibility and all-round bad taste and this American story was immediately picked up by the world press, eager to disseminate the great news of the conquest of tuberculosis with scant regard for the full facts and the possible future implications.

The very advantages which made isoniazid attractive were those which gave most cause for concern to physicians already experienced in the use of streptomycin and P.A.S. It was obviously potent, was easily administered, had a low incidence of toxicity and, above all, was relatively inexpensive—all factors which combined to make it a tempting drug to prescribe, especially for treatment outside hospital. Its widespread use within a short period of time was thus to be anticipated and the perils inherent in any such universal and precipitate employment were obvious. The problem of drug resistance in particular required intensive study and the British Medical Research Council asked their Tuberculosis Chemotherapy Trials Committee to put in train immediately the organization of a controlled trial.

17   Robitzek, E. H. & Selikoff, I. J. (1952) Hydrazine derivative of isonicotinic acid (Rimifon, Marsalid) in the treatment of acute progressive caseous-pneumonic tuberculosis. A preliminary report. *Am. Rev. Tuberc.* 65. 402.

In this trial the efficacy of isoniazid was measured against that of the best known chemotherapy (streptomycin and P.A.S.) and the previous routine of random allocation of patients to their treatment group was followed. Furthermore, in view of the special features of isoniazid and the uninhibited publicity which it had already attracted, the Committee considered it essential that reliable information regarding its efficiency should be released as soon as it became available and accordingly the trial was designed to permit a continuing analysis of the accumulating data, thus enabling important results to be reported without delay.

The trial began in March 1952 and an interim report was issued in October summarizing the findings to date.

> The conclusion, judging wholly from short-term results, is that isoniazid is a very effective drug in pulmonary tuberculosis, but given alone it is not more effective than streptomycin plus P.A.S. Bacillary resistance to isoniazid was found in 11% of cases at the end of the first month, in 52% at the end of the second, and in 71% at the end of the trial. Lack of progress, as assessed by radiological change, was found to be related to the emergence of drug resistance. This is therefore a most serious problem affecting the use of isoniazid.[18]

There was soon ample evidence from American and other sources to corroborate the Medical Research Council's findings and to dispel the illusion, still cherished by a few supreme optimists, that isoniazid could on its own solve the world's tuberculosis problem. The disappointment felt over the remarkable rapidity with which bacillary resistence developed when the drug was used singly was, however, tempered by the realization that it was likely to play an important part in any programme of combined therapy and its value in this role became the subject of the next series of British trials. By 1953 it had been established that a daily dose of 20 g P.A.S. with 200 mg isoniazid was of the same order of effectiveness as streptomycin 1 g daily with isoniazid 200 gm daily and as streptomycin 1 g daily with P.A.S. 20 g daily. An attempt to vary the dosages of streptomycin and P.A.S. while maintaining the isoniazid constant at 200 mg daily was now indicated. Four different regimens were selected and by February 1955 the Committee had accumulated sufficient evidence to justify a further report to the Council.

18 Medical Research Council Investigation (1952) The treatment of pulmonary tuberculosis with isoniazid. An interim report. *Br. med. J.* 2, 735.

It is concluded, *judging solely from the results at three months*, that strepto-mycin 1 g daily plus isoniazid 200 mg daily is not only the most effective of the four treatments but represents the most effective drug combination studied at any stage of the trial. Streptomycin 1 g twice a week plus isoniazid 200 mg daily is less satisfactory in preventing the emergence of streptomycin-resistant organisms, and its use as a primary chemo-therapeutic measure cannot be recommended. P.A.S. plus isoniazid has proved itself a very effective combination of drugs although it is not quite so powerful as daily streptomycin plus isoniazid. There is little to choose between the clinical and bacteriological efficacy of 20 g and 10 g P.A.S. (sodium salt) daily plus isoniazid 200 mg daily. Either combina-tion of P.A.S. with isoniazid is a most valuable oral form of combined chemotherapy in the treatment of pulmonary tuberculosis.[19]

The evidence which had been accumulated during the course of this trial, showing the remarkable manner in which isoniazid could enhance a chemotherapeutic combination, proved to be the starting point for the most complete re-appraisal and re-orientation of ideas on treatment that had so far taken place throughout the centuries-old history of the disease. The possibilities inherent in a programme of long-term combined chemotherapy were at first visualized only by a very few. Indeed such a distinguished scientist as Georges Canetti, director of the laboratory of the Pasteur Institute, was writing in 1955 that

Short of spectacular progress in one way or another, it is unlikely that chemotherapy will become the exclusive treatment of pulmonary tuberculosis. There are too many factors against it, . . . Most important among them is the existence of caseous necrosis with its numerous effects upon bacterial growth. As things are at present, chemotherapy cannot suffice for the treatment of tuberculosis unless the diagnosis can be established before caseation occurs. Such a clinical revolution is out of the question.[20]

But even before Canetti's book had left the printing press clinical opinion had begun to change and, within a relatively brief period, long-term combined chemotherapy had emerged as the sole treat-ment necessary for the achievement of complete cure in uncomplicated

19 Medical Research Council Investigation (1955) Various combinations of isoniazid with streptomycin or with P.A.S. in the treatment of pulmonary tuberculosis. *Br. med. J.* *1*, 435.
20 Canetti, G. (1955) *The Tubercle Bacillus in the Pulmonary Lesion of Man.* p. 205. New York: Springer.

cases of either pulmonary or extrapulmonary disease. In Britain the chief architects of this revolutionary approach were those working in the Edinburgh school led by Professor John Crofton. Crofton, a member of the Medical Research Council's Trials Committee, had been quick to appreciate the full significance of the information which the trials were producing and, once it had become clear that the use of combined chemotherapy could virtually abolish the spectre of drug resistance, he and his colleagues made its employment their routine clinical practice. Shortly afterwards, and confident that their action would be justified by results, they began extending the duration of the treatment to cover much longer periods than the three months on which the trial findings had been based. The introduction of this policy was eased by a coincidental reorganization of the Edinburgh tuberculosis service resulting in the allocation of both clinic and hospital duties to each of the senior physicians, an arrangement which ensured that the individual patient remained under the care of the same physician from notification until final discharge. Thus not only was a good chemotherapy regime guaranteed but the continuity of supervision did much to ensure the co-operation of the patient in actually taking the drugs—a co-operation which too many physicians were tending to take too much for granted.

The results of this policy were prompt and impressive, being reflected in a low mortality rate and also in a low relapse rate among the survivors. Such deaths as did occur were largely attributable to drug-resistance acquired before admission or to admission in a moribund condition, while the relapse rate was also linked to drug-resistance and, significantly, to the duration of chemotherapy. Thus in one group of 63 patients whose bacilli were fully sensitive and who had received more than 18 months continuous chemotherapy there had been no relapses. In reporting the results the Edinburgh team wrote:

> We consider that the weapons now available are sufficient to command recovery in nearly all newly diagnosed cases of pulmonary tuberculosis. One hundred per cent success is not an unreasonable target. Failure can almost always be traced to errors committed by the doctor or by the patient, the doctor failing to prescribe reliable combinations of drugs or the patient failing to take his drugs as prescribed.[21]

The conclusions reached in this publication were reinforced one year later when Crofton, addressing a plenary session of the British

21 Ross, J. D. et al. (1958) Hospital treatment of pulmonary tuberculosis. *Br. med. J.* 1, 237.

Medical Association at Birmingham, declared that 'the right use of modern methods of chemotherapy now makes it possible to aim at 100% success in the treatment of pulmonary tuberculosis'.[22] But in making this declaration he was careful to emphasize that

> such results are attainable only by exercising the greatest care in prescribing the right combination of drugs, by handling the patient so that he continues to take his chemotherapy conscientiously over long periods of time, during much of which he is feeling perfectly well, and by carrying out the most careful drug-resistance tests in those in whom there is any reason to suspect that drug resistance may have occurred. The slightest error on the part of either doctor or patient may result in disaster. In no disease is the result of conscientious doctoring more rewarding. In none is the result of carelessness or ignorance more tragic for the patient.

By 1959, then, the principles which should govern the effective chemotherapy of tuberculosis had been clearly established and when these were applied rigorously the results proved to be all that the Edinburgh workers had claimed. Thus the team of physicians who staffed the tuberculosis service of the large industrial city of Birmingham were able to report in 1960 that of 530 newly diagnosed patients admitted to hospital between 1 January 1957 and 31 December 1958, whose bacilli on admission were sensitive to at least two of the main antituberculosis drugs, all had achieved sputum conversion on chemotherapy alone.[23]

Similar results were not reproduced universally since in order to obtain such figures a high degree of dedication and enthusiasm was required from the physicians while the maximum co-operation of the patient was essential. In an imperfect world neither of these criteria were met on each and every occasion, but, in spite of lapses, the overall impact of modern chemotherapy was sufficient to produce a dramatic fall in the national death-rate accompanied by a less dramatic but nonetheless undeniable reduction in the number of new cases. As a natural sequel to these remarkable happenings many queries had already been raised about the role of such traditional aspects of tuberculosis treatment as bed-rest, sanatoria and rehabilitation centres while in some quarters it was even being suggested that the preliminary period of hospital treatment, so far regarded as essential for

22 Crofton, J. (1959) Chemotherapy of pulmonary tuberculosis. *Br. med. J. 1*, 1610.
23 Thomas, H. E. et al. (1960) 100% sputum conversion in newly diagnosed pulmonary tuberculosis. *Br. med. J. 2*, 1185.

the initiation of chemotherapy, had become an unnecessary refinement which could readily be discarded without detriment to the patient and his family. The problem of the drug-resistant case, nightmare of both physician and of public health specialist, continued to cause concern and the search for further antibacterial agents which could either replace or supplement the existing drugs was being pursued with energy and determination even if with only limited success.

But, while the utilization of modern chemotherapy presented no really insuperable problems to those nations with an organized tuberculosis service backed by adequate financial resources, the position was vastly different in the undeveloped tropical countries. Here the need was great but invariably the national budget was unable to sustain even the most modest programme of chemotherapy, both through lack of hospital accommodation and of trained personnel as well as through sheer inability to meet the cost of the drugs. Salvation in such a situation appeared to depend on the discovery of another drug possessing the attributes of isoniazid—high efficacy and low cost—with which the latter could be paired, and also on confirmation of the germinating idea that hospital admission was not necessarily a prerequisite for effective treatment. Research programmes aimed at resolving these problems were mounted in the 1950s and the results were coming in during the first half of the next decade. These projects not only produced results of value to the undeveloped countries on whose behalf they had originally been launched, but the findings held lessons also for those amongst the sophisticated nations of the western world who were not too proud to make the necessary adjustments in their own national programmes.

Chapter Nineteen
The 'Reserve' Drugs

Gratification at the results which were being achieved by the use of 'standard' chemotherapy, as the triple regimen of streptomycin, P.A.S. and isoniazid came to be termed, was never allowed to over-shadow the apprehension with which drug resistance was regarded nor to obscure the need to provide a solution to this problem. The ideal answer, of course, was to ensure by perfect initial treatment that drug resistance did not develop; but the attainment of this ideal was only possible in the complete absence of any of the usual human frailties in both physician and patient. Since the achievement of such a Utopian situation was highly improbable there began an intensive hunt for further antimicrobial agents with the hunters ever hopeful that by casting widely another isoniazid might eventually emerge. But while there was no lack of antibacterial agents with some de-monstrable activity against *M. tuberculosis* only a few had the qualities to make them acceptable as a 'second best' in the face of resistance to one or more of the drugs used in initial therapy: these few came to be grouped together under the blanket title of 'reserve' drugs.

An early and important member of the group was thioacetazone, a thiosemicarbazone which was first introduced for the treatment of tuberculosis by Domagk.[1] While there was good evidence that thioacetazone possessed antituberculosis activity approximately equal to that of P.A.S. there was concern about its toxicity and, following a report by Hinshaw and Walsh McDermott,[2] enthusiasm for its use waned until in 1952 it was almost totally extinguished on the intro-duction of isoniazid. Thioacetazone became the centre of renewed interest in 1960 due primarily to the urgent need for an effective yet

1 Domagk, G. (1950) Investigations on the antituberculous activity of the thiosemi-carbazones *in vitro* and *in vivo*. *Am. Rev. Tuberc.* *61*, 8.
2 Hinshaw, H. C. & McDermott, W. (1950) Thiosemicarbazone therapy of tuberculosis in humans. *Am. Rev. Tuberc.* *61*, 145.

inexpensive agent to be used as a companion drug to isoniazid in countries with a high incidence of tuberculosis allied to a low budget. It was attractively cheap and was accordingly tested for therapeutic reliability in a well-planned investigation in East Africa, a trial which convincingly demonstrated that isoniazid, 300 mg and thioacetazone, 150 mg, provided an effective daily regimen without—at least as far as East Africa was concerned—any prohibitive degree of toxicity[3]: this combination was thereafter adopted as the basic regimen throughout that area. Other countries with a similar socio-economic structure endeavoured to follow the East African example but some encountered an incidence of side-effects high enough to make the drug unacceptable. A suggestion that racial differences might be an operative factor in this varying pattern of toxicity prompted an extensive trial, organized by the British Medical Research Council's Tuberculosis Research Unit, which involved 13 different countries, widely distributed throughout the world, from Europe through Asia Minor, Africa and India to the Pacific and the Far East. The result of this trial was reported in 1966 with the following conclusion:

> This investigation has shown that there has been a total level of side-effects associated with the use of thioacetazone which is acceptable in the socio-economic circumstances in which therapy is undertaken in most developing countries ... However, the study has also suggested that both the incidence and the nature of the side-effects may vary sufficiently from country to country fully to support the recommendations of the 1964 WHO Expert Committee that 'whenever it is decided to use isoniazid plus thioacetazone on a wide scale in a community for the first time, it is essential first to undertake a careful investigation of the toxicity of the regimen in an adequate number of cases'.[4]

Apart from those areas and countries where cost was of paramount importance there was no inclination to revert to thioacetazone, and when a substitute for the standard regimen was necessary reliance was placed on a selection made from the ever-widening range of 'reserve' drugs which were becoming available.

Prominent among these was pyrazinamide which was originally synthesized in the Lederle Laboratories. Animal experiments were encouraging and a clinical trial by Yeager, Munroe and Dessau

3 East Africa/British Medical Research Council Second Thioacetazone Investigation (1963) Isoniazid with thioacetazone in the treatment of pulmonary tuberculosis in East Africa. *Tubercle 44*, 301.
4 Miller, A. B., Fox, W. & Tall, R. (1966) An international co-operative investigation into thiacetazone (thioacetazone) side-effects. *Tubercle 47*, 33.

indicated that pyrazinamide had considerable potency as an anti-tuberculosis agent but with the inevitable drawback—resistant strains of bacilli emerged with remarkable rapidity when the drug was given alone.[5] Attention had already been directed by McCune and Thompsett to the unique effect of pyrazinamide combined with isoniazid on mice infected with tuberculosis where the combination appeared to eradicate all bacilli from the spleen.[6] A clinical trial of these two drugs was begun by Walsh McDermott and a number of associates and in 1954 they reported in the following terms:

> It is concluded that pyrazinamide–isoniazid exercises antituberculous activity *in vivo* of a sort superior to that of the other current antituberculous drugs used either singly or together. Moreover, the animal studies indicate that the antimicrobial action of pyrazinamide–isoniazid is not only quantitively superior but is qualitatively unique among anti-tuberculous chemotherapies. It is further concluded, however, that the high incidence of hepatitis in man during pyrazinamide–isoniazid administration makes the use of this regimen in present dosage inadvisable as a treatment of tuberculosis.[7]

The threat of hepatotoxicity exercised a restraining influence on any enthusiasm for pyrazinamide: with careful dosage the risk could be reduced but even in the most favourable circumstances it was necessary to monitor liver function closely with appropriate tests at approximately fortnightly intervals. As the number of patients willing to submit to such a programme was limited pyrazinamide fell out of favour and remained so for some 15 years until changing concepts in regard to chemotherapy brought it to the fore again.

Ethionamide was introduced into clinical practice in 1959 when, following a series of experimental studies by Rist, Grumbach and Libermann,[8] Brouet and a group of colleagues carried out a trial at the Hospital Cochin in Paris and reported that

> The result obtained when the thioamide was used in multiple-drug regimens, including isoniazid and isoniazid and streptomycin, were considered to be most satisfactory . . . When used in association with other drugs, the thioamide has brought about considerable improvement of

5   Yeager, R. L., Munroe, W. G. C. & Dessau, F. I. (1952) Pyrazinamide (aldinamide) in the treatment of pulmonary tuberculosis. *Am. Rev. Tuberc. 65*, 523.

6   McCune, R. & Thompsett, R. Quoted by McDermott W. et al. (1954) Pyrazinamide-isoniazid in tuberculosis. *Am. Rev. Tuberc. 69*, 319.

7   McDermott, W. et al. (1954) Pyrazinamide–isoniazid in tuberculosis. *Am. Rev. Tuberc. 69*, 319.

8   Rist, N., Grumbach, F. & Libermann, D. (1959) Experiments in the antituberculous activity of alpha-ethyl-thioisonicotinamide. *Am. Rev. Tuberc. 79*, 1.

the lesions and reversal of infectiousness in patients who had received much previous therapy but whose strain of tubercle bacilli were completely resistant *in vitro* to isoniazid and to streptomycin.[9]

It was unfortunate that ethionamide was endowed with unpleasant side-effects which were reflected chiefly in the gastrointestinal tract with anorexia, nausea and vomiting as prominent features. The optimum dose was considered to be 1 g daily but this was more than the majority of patients were prepared to tolerate and it was usually necessary to compromise at 0.75 g although, even at this level, tolerance was frequently stretched to the limit.

Other preparations joining the list of 'reserve' drugs included three further antibiotics: viomycin, cycloserine and capreomycin. None was particularly potent and all had appreciable toxicity but nevertheless for a time they represented the only answer to drug resistance. When resistance was confined to one, or even two, of the standard agents the situation was usually controllable; but when all three were involved (fortunately a relatively rare occurrence), and reliance had to be placed entirely on 'reserve' drugs, the position became critical. To juggle successfully with a minimum of three potentially toxic products required constant and vigilant supervision by the physician together with maximum co-operation from the patient who, in his own interests as well as those of the community, had to be coaxed into persevering with an unpleasant and seemingly endless regimen. In such circumstances it was little wonder that resistance to standard chemotherapy was dreaded as posing one of the most difficult problems in the therapy of the disease.

The first suggestion that better things might be on the way appeared about 1962 when ethambutol, another new drug developed by the Lederle Laboratories, showed some signs of promise. Initial experiments both *in vitro* and *in vivo* were sufficiently encouraging to justify clinical trials and by 1966 Donomae and Yamamoto were able to report that

> treatment with this drug was found to be especially effective in producing negative conversion in a high degree soon after the institution of treatment. Used in adequate doses, this drug showed only a low incidence of side-effects. On the basis of these findings, ethambutol may be regarded as an excellent antituberculous agent.[10]

9 Brouet, G. et al. (1959) Observations on the antituberculous effectiveness of alpha-ethyl-thioisonicotinamide in humans. *Am. Rev. Tuberc.* 79, 6.

10 Donomae, I. & Yamamoto, K. (1966) Clinical evaluation of ethambutol in pulmonary tuberculosis, *Ann. N.Y. Acad. Sci. 135*, 849.

Subsequent work confirmed the early reports though it became clear that the action of ethambutol was bacteriostatic rather than bactericidal and that its main use would probably be as a replacement for P.A.S. when the latter was being badly tolerated. It enjoyed two distinct advantages in that it was easily administered and relatively non-toxic. The main manifestation of toxicity was retrobulbar neuritis but this was uncommon when the correct dosage was used and the damage was almost always completely reversed when the drug was withdrawn. It appeared therefore that ethambutol was likely to be an important addition to the 'reserve' list and that, like thioacetazone, it had a distinct chance of later promotion to the ranks of standard chemotherapy.

Research in this huge field had still to yield its greatest prize. In 1966 a new family of antibiotics, the rifamycins, emerged into the light of day. These were semi-synthetic compounds which had been developed in the Lepetit Research Laboratories from *Streptomyces mediterranei* and the first which was made available for trial, rifamycin SV, showed a high degree of antituberculosis activity *in vitro*.[11] Its pharmacological properties were such that an adequate serum level could only be attained by intravenous injection, a defect which provided the stimulus necessary for the development of rifamycin AMP, better known as rifampicin (rifampin in the United States), which, given by mouth, was readily absorbed to produce a high serum level. Rifampicin was shown to be markedly bactericidal, approaching in its *in vitro* effect the action of isoniazid, a finding confirmed by animal experiments indicating that it was as effective as isoniazid in mice and as streptomycin in guinea-pigs. The work was taken a stage further by Grumbach who carried out *in vivo* studies of capreomycin, ethambutol and rifampicin and concluded:

> This experimental investigation of three new drugs has shown that the therapeutic value of rifampicin is certainly greatly superior to that of the other two, capreomycin and ethambutol. It is also superior to that of isoniazid. The discovery of rifampicin appears to open a new era in antituberculous chemotherapy.[12]

The favourable opinion expressed by Grumbach was confirmed by a

11 Füresz, S. & Timball, M. T. (1963) Antibacterial activity of rifamycins. *Chemotherapia* 7, 200.
12 Grumbach, F. (1969) Experimental *in vivo* studies of new antituberculosis drugs. Supplement to *Tubercle 50*, 12.

number of clinical reports appearing in 1971, 1972 and 1974[13, 14, 15] all recording highly satisfactory results in patients, resistant to standard chemotherapy, who had had rifampicin added to their reserve drug regimen.

The introduction of two new drugs, one of which had been shown to be highly bactericidal, naturally caused questioning glances to be cast at the established triad of streptomycin, P.A.S. and isoniazid. There seemed much to be said for the replacement of P.A.S. which, with its unpleasant side-effects, was generally held, rightly or wrongly, to be an important cause of failure in patient co-operation. Ethambutol, by comparison, was largely devoid of troublesome accompaniments and had the additional advantage that it could be taken in a single daily dose. An extensive controlled trial under the auspices of the United States Public Health Service investigated its use in initial therapy and came to the conclusion that ethambutol in a dose of 15 mg per kg was therapeutically an effective substitute for P.A.S. and was virtually non-toxic.[16]

Even as ethambutol was being accepted into the fold the evidence accumulating on rifampicin was showing that another antibacterial agent of major importance had been discovered, one that, on grounds of therapeutic efficiency alone and disregarding its relative freedom from unpleasant side-effects, must have a strong claim for inclusion amongst the drugs used in initial therapy. The claim of this newcomer was strengthened by a further United States Public Health Service trial which, organized on similar lines to that employed to investigate ethambutol, reported in the most favourable terms that 'rifampin is a well tolerated oral drug that when taken in combination with isoniazid is more effective than the best multidrug regimen previously used for far-advanced cavitary disease'.[17]

Unfortunately there was one important factor which militated

13 Somner, A. R. et al. (1971) Drug resistant pulmonary tuberculosis treated with ethambutol and rifampicin in North East England. *Tubercle 52*, 266.

14 Aquinas, M. & Citron, K. M. (1972) Rifampicin, ethambutol and capreomycin in pulmonary tuberculosis, previously treated with both first and second line drugs: the results of 2 years chemotherapy. *Tubercle 53*, 153.

15 Andrews, R. H. et al. (1974) Treatment of isoniazid resistant pulmonary tuberculosis with ethambutol, rifampicin and capreomycin: A co-operative study in England and Wales. *Tubercle 55*, 105.

16 Doster, B. et al. (1973) USPHS Therapy Trials: Ethambutol in the initial treatment of pulmonary tuberculosis. *Am. Rev. resp. Dis. 2*, 177.

17 Newman, R. et al. (1974) USPHS Therapy Trials: Rifampin in initial treatment of pulmonary tuberculosis. *Am. Rev. resp. Dis. 2*, 216.

against the immediate incorporation of rifampicin into initial treatment—expense. A leading article in *Tubercle* stressed this inhibiting
factor.

> It is a highly expensive drug and seems likely to remain so. In many
> countries the cost will be prohibitive. It will be far more important to put
> the available resources to better use by improving primary treatment
> with the cheaper regimens . . . In Great Britain there seems no justifica-
> tion for using rifampicin at present in initial treatment except in the rare
> cases of severe intolerance to PAS or toxicity to streptomycin.[18]

Later exploration of the therapeutic properties of rifampicin was to
reveal that its unique bactericidal action against *M. tuberculosis* might
in certain circumstances offset at least part of its extra cost. In the
meantime its discovery, together with that of ethambutol, had ensured that effective and acceptable alternatives were now available to
cope with the problem of resistance to the standard drugs—a happier
situation which brought a sense of relief to physicians which only
those who had had to struggle with the earlier 'reserve' drugs could
appreciate to the full.

18   Leading Article (1969) Rifampicin. *Tubercle* 50, 318.

Chapter Twenty
The Madras Experiment
and its Sequelae

By the early 1960s the treatment of the newly diagnosed case of pulmonary tuberculosis had become a standard procedure and followed a standard pattern, at least as far as Europe and North America were concerned. With the possibility of primary drug resistance ever in mind it was customary to initiate treatment with all three main drugs, continuing this triple therapy until the results of pre-treatment sputum sensitivity tests became available: at this stage, if the organisms proved to be fully sensitive, streptomycin might be withdrawn and treatment continued with P.A.S. and isoniazid alone. As a general rule patients were admitted to hospital for treatment and discharge was not considered until the first negative sputum culture had been produced. This pattern, while fairly generally practised, was not in any way rigid and variations both in the duration of the triple drug regimen and of in-patient treatment were at the discretion of the physician—a discretion not always uniformly exercised.

Doubts regarding the optimum duration of treatment, with opinion ranging from a minimum of 12 months up to a lifetime sentence,[1] had been largely resolved following the Medical Research Council's report on a trial designed for that specific purpose. The results of this trial, which were expressed in terms of bacteriological relapse, showed that stopping treatment after only six months was penalized by a rate as high as 62 per cent. Carrying on for a further six months reduced the percentage of relapses to 19 while a total of two years' treatment yielded better results still with the very low rate of 4 per cent. Other findings emerging from this trial were that no worthwhile benefit resulted from continuing chemotherapy for a third year and that those patients who had had their P.A.S. and

---

1 Dooneief, A. S., Hite, K. E. & Bloch, R. G. (1955) Indefinitely prolonged chemotherapy for tuberculosis. *Archs intern. Med.* *96*, 470.

isoniazid (the regimen on which the trial had been based) supplemented during the first six weeks by daily streptomycin derived a significant advantage.[2]

While this pattern of hospital admission, with an initial period on a triple drug schedule followed by oral therapy until a total of two years treatment had been completed, presented no real problem to the affluent nations whose level of expenditure was dictated by the requirements of the situation rather than by what the country could afford, there were large areas of the world which presented a vastly different problem. In the jargon of the age the technologically advanced countries (the 'haves') could readily afford what was miles beyond the reach of the developing countries (the 'have-nots') yet the needs of the latter were very great for they carried the burden of a severe tuberculosis problem allied to a very low national budget. Not for them the elaborate tuberculosis control programmes with local clinics, adequate laboratory services, mass radiography units and plentiful sanatorium beds which Europe and North America had come to regard as essential. If they were to have the benefits of chemotherapy then a completely new approach must be planned, an approach in which simplicity and frugality could be combined without an undue sacrifice of efficiency. Fox put the matter in stark perspective when he wrote that 'The actual cost of the drugs in antituberculosis regimens is an important consideration in developing countries where the total expenditure on all the health services is often of the order of 4s per head of population per year.'[3]

As the full possibilities of chemotherapy became apparent the idea that sanatorium admission might not necessarily be a prerequisite for adequate treatment began to germinate and those preoccupied with tuberculosis as a world problem realized that, if admission could be shown to be unnecessary, a major obstacle would have been cleared from their path. Such an hypothesis had to be put to the test and in 1956 a research project, designed for this specific purpose, was launched with the opening of the Tuberculosis Chemotherapy Centre in Madras. The Centre, under the joint auspices of the Indian Council of Medical Research, the Madras State Government, the World Health Organisation and the British Medical Research Council,

2 British Medical Research Council (1962) Long-term chemotherapy in the treatment of chronic pulmonary tuberculosis with cavitation. *Tubercle 43*, 201.
3 Fox, W. (1970) Advances in the treatment of respiratory tuberculosis. *Practitioner 205*, 502.

was charged with the task of conducting controlled clinical investigations which would provide information on the home treatment of pulmonary tuberculosis by chemotherapy. 'This was a problem of great importance since at that time there were only 23 000 beds for tuberculosis in the whole country with an estimated 1.5 million infectious cases.'[4]

The first investigation which was planned and executed was destined to become a classic and to establish the Centre firmly in the international league as a source of meticulous reliable work, the results of which could be accepted with total confidence. This pioneer trial set out to compare the results of treatment in two groups of patients: one group was treated in a sanatorium and the other group at home, 'home' in this context usually meaning an overcrowded hovel in the poorest quarter of Madras, but each group received the same chemotherapy consisting of daily P.A.S. and isoniazid given for a period of one year. The limit of one year was imposed since it was considered to be unrealistic to continue for a longer period in a country with very limited financial resources. All patients involved in the trial were followed up for five years, in itself a tribute to the dedicated work of the Centre team and to the feat of organization which enabled such a project to be carried through to finality. At the conclusion of the five-year period 90 per cent of the patients treated at home and 89 per cent of those initially in a sanatorium had bacteriologically quiescent disease as indicated by consistently negative sputum cultures over a period of from 54 to 60 months.[5]

This admirable work comprized the main investigation but during its conduct there were opportunities to study two associated problems the reports on which constituted useful by-products. The first concerned the fate of contacts, an aspect of the trial which had been a source of some anxiety during the planning stage though in the event it became apparent that domiciliary treatment had not increased the risk to contacts within the family circle.[6] The trial had also provided an excellent opportunity to study the role of diet in treatment: while

4 Indian Council of Medical Research (1967) *Tuberculosis Chemotherapy Centre, Madras. A review of research activities 1956–1966.* p. 1. New Delhi.

5 Dawson, J. J. Y. et al. (1966) A 5-year study of patients with pulmonary tuberculosis in a concurrent comparison of home and sanatorium treatment for one year with isoniazid and P.A.S. *Bull. Wld. Hlth. Org. 34*, 533.

6 Kamat, S. R. et al. (1966) A controlled study of the influence of segregation of tuberculous patients for one year on the attack rate of tuberculosis in a 5-year study of close family contacts in South India. *Bull. Wld. Hlth. Org. 34*, 517.

the sanatorium-treated patients received a nutritionally adequate and well-balanced diet, those treated entirely at home subsisted on the classical South Indian diet, deficient in total calories, fats, proteins, minerals and vitamins, and adequate only in its carbohydrate content. The evidence was encouraging and re-assuring for, as the trial proceeded, it became clear that diet contributed little to the response to treatment and had no influence on the liability to relapse[7]—the most sacred of all the sacred cows in the therapy of tuberculosis had at last been slaughtered.

The work at Madras continued, other aspects of chemotherapy were investigated and the papers published from the Centre continued to bear the hallmark of quality and authority. Eight years after its opening what had originally been intended as a project of limited scope and duration had proved of such value that in 1964 the Centre was made a permanent establishment under the Indian Council of Medical Research with a Project Committee, which included representatives of the World Health Organisation and the British Medical Research Council, to guide the research.

The facets of chemotherapy investigated at the Centre were many and varied but among the most important was one—the self-administration of drugs—which had invariably bedevilled *all* oral medication and which was now causing much concern in the management of tuberculosis. Even though treatment might be initiated in hospital it required to be continued for months on an out-patient basis when the daily administration of the drugs was in the individual's own hands—and evidence was accumulating which showed that irregularity in such self-administration was a disconcertingly frequent occurrence. Most workers were inclined to lay the main blame for this at the door of P.A.S. with its notoriously unpleasant accompaniments but an extensive study of the subject at Madras revealed a wider picture.

> The studies at the Madras Centre have shown that self-administration is a problem, not only with a mixture of P.A.S. and isoniazid, but also with isoniazid by itself and even with a placebo. It is a problem with cachets and with tablets, whether large or small, and with a single tablet daily as well as when several are prescribed daily, whether this is as one

---

7 Ramakrishnan, C. V. et al. (1961) The role of diet in the treatment of pulmonary tuberculosis. An evaluation in a controlled chemotherapy study in home and sanatorium patients in South India. *Bull. Wld. Hlth. Org. 25*, 339.

dose a day or two doses a day. Even a year of supervised administration in sanatorium does not avoid subsequent irregularity.[8]

While a variety of causes were noted as contributing to the irregularity, two stood out above all others—forgetfulness and sheer indolence, a finding which was supported in several studies carried out in Britain.

Recognition of the existence of this problem on a wide scale constituted a challenge. Various methods had been devised for the detection of irregularity but its elimination demanded something more than mere reproof and exhortation, and the only solution which seemed likely to be effective would be one which would transfer the responsibility for the medication from the patient to the clinic staff. Such a solution would present formidable problems of organization so long as it involved daily out-patient attendance or the daily administration of treatment to the patient in his own home and would clearly be impractical in most areas. A discovery made in Madras during the course of work on the metabolism of isoniazid was to provide a scientific basis for an alternative approach. Hitherto the dosage of all antituberculosis chemotherapy had been aimed at the maintenance of a constant minimum inhibitory serum level but this hypothesis was now called in question when it was shown by the Madras workers that the therapeutic response to isoniazid was related to the peak concentration attained in the serum rather than to the duration of time for which an inhibitory level was maintained.[9] This finding provided an argument for giving the daily requirement of isoniazid as one single dose instead of the usual divided doses but it went further still by causing consideration to be given to the possibility of a fully intermittent regimen in which a high dose of isoniazid would play an essential part.

A clinical trial was planned in which streptomycin 1 g and an oral dose of isoniazid calculated to provide 14 mg per kg body weight were given together under supervision twice weekly. This treatment was continued for one year and proved highly effective, probably more so than the standard oral P.A.S. and isoniazid given daily to the control group, though the difference fell just short of attaining

8 Fox, W. (1962) Self-administration of medicaments. *Bull. int. Un. Tuberc. 32*, 307.
9 Tuberculosis Chemotherapy Centre, Madras (1960) A concurrent comparison of isoniazid plus P.A.S. with three regimens of isoniazid alone in the domiciliary treatment of pulmonary tuberculosis in South India. *Bull. Wld. Hlth. Org. 23*, 535.

statistical significance.[10] Follow-up study two years later showed a slightly lower relapse rate in the recipients of the intermittent regimen while it was noted that, of the five patients on that regimen who were so unlucky as to relapse, four did so with fully sensitive organisms.[11] The logical deduction from this finding was that the relapses occurred because the period of treatment was too short and that continuance of the treatment beyond one year could well have resulted in a negligible relapse rate.[12]

Unfortunately the conditions which contributed to the success of supervised intermittent chemotherapy in Madras and in out-patient practice in Britain[13] could not be reproduced satisfactorily in many of the overseas areas where supervision was most required. The most excellent intentions were defeated by problems of organization and it became necessary to think again.

Wallace Fox, director of the British Medical Research Council's Tuberculosis Unit, who had been closely involved with affairs in Madras and with numerous other overseas research projects, had long held the view that top priority in chemotherapeutic research should be given to the discovery of some means of reducing the total duration of treatment. Starting with the premise that the duration of chemotherapy was the prime factor contributing to its premature termination and being convinced that it was psychologically undesirable for even a symptom-free patient to feel that he was suffering from and receiving treatment for a disease over such a long period of time, he had gone on 'to consider the value of concentrating resources and facilities on a period of chemotherapy shorter than the minimum of one year'.[14]

The introduction of rifampicin with its obvious potency and special bactericidal activity seemed an indication that the time had come to attempt another break with tradition and accordingly a large-scale,

10 Tuberculosis Chemotherapy Centre, Madras (1964) A concurrent comparison of intermittent (twice-weekly) isoniazid plus streptomycin and daily isoniazid plus P.A.S. in the domiciliary treatment of pulmonary tuberculosis. *Bull. Wld Hlth Org. 31*, 247.

11 Nazareth, O. et al. (1966) A two-year follow-up of patients with quiescent pulmonary tuberculosis following a year of chemotherapy with an intermittent (twice-weekly) regimen of isoniazid plus streptomycin or a daily regimen of isoniazid plus P.A.S. *Tubercle 47*, 178.

12 Fox, W. (1968) The John Barnwell Lecture. Changing concepts in the chemotherapy of pulmonary tuberculosis. *Am. Rev. resp. Dis. 97*, 767.

13 Poole, G. W. & Stradling, P. (1965) The long-term use of intermittent streptomycin plus isoniazid in the treatment of tuberculosis. *Tubercle 46*, 290.

14 Fox, W. & Mitchison, D. A. (1975) Short-course chemotherapy for pulmonary tuberculosis. *Am. Rev. resp. Dis. 111*, 325.

co-operative, controlled clinical study was set up in East Africa and Zambia, in association with the East African Tuberculosis Investigation Centre, to explore the possibilities of short-course chemotherapy. The patients admitted to the trial, newly diagnosed cases with positive sputa and extensive, cavitated disease, were allocated by random selection to one of four treatment regimens of six months duration. Each regimen contained streptomycin and isoniazid but three had, in addition, another drug—either rifampicin, pyrazinamide or thioacetazone. All drugs were given daily and the results were compared with those obtained by standard treatment of eighteen months duration. The inclusion of pyrazinamide in one of the regimens under trial reflected a recent revival of interest in this drug which, on its first appearance in the 1950s, had, in combination with isoniazid, revealed remarkable antituberculosis activity in animal experiments. Fear of toxicity had restricted its employment in clinical practice but, with careful dosage, this fear proved to have been exaggerated and apart from its undoubted potency pyrazinamide enjoyed an additional advantage in being appreciably cheaper than rifampicin.

Assessment after six months' treatment showed that all the regimens had been uniformly and highly effective but in the subsequent follow-up period sharp differences appeared. Bacteriological relapse occurred in 18 per cent of the streptomycin-isoniazid group and in 21 per cent of those who had also received thioacetazone while with the regimens containing either rifampicin or pyrazinamide the relapse rates were 4 per cent and 6 per cent respectively. Most of the relapses occurred in the three months following cessation of treatment and practically all the patients concerned produced organisms still fully sensitive.[15] Further study confirmed the efficacy of the rifampicin and pyrazinamide combinations: at the end of 30 months follow-up the relapses in the two groups were 3 per cent and 8 per cent, a finding which appeared to justify fully the claim by the authors of these comprehensive reports that 'short-course chemotherapy constitutes a development of major importance in the treatment of tuberculosis'.[16]

Interest in short-course chemotherapy now became universal for even the affluent nations were sufficiently cost-conscious to ap-

15 East African/British Medical Research Councils (1972) Controlled clinical trial of short-course (6 months) regimens of chemotherapy for treatment of pulmonary tuberculosis. *Lancet i*, 1079.
16 *Ibid.* (1974) *Lancet ii*, 1975.

preciate that curtailment of the period of treatment, if it could be accomplished successfully, was economically desirable both from the national and the individual viewpoints. A trial was reported in France in 1974[17] while in Brazil Poppe de Figueiredo and his colleagues reported on a pilot trial at the 22nd International Tuberculosis Conference in 1973.[18] The Research Committee of the British Thoracic and Tuberculosis Association, engaged on a similar project, reported highly favourable results from a combination of isoniazid and rifampicin supplemented during the first two months by either ethambutol or streptomycin. One group of patients who received therapy for 6 months were, with a single exception, culture-negative at the conclusion of treatment but had a 5 per cent relapse rate during the following 18 months. By contrast a group receiving treatment for 9 months all converted successfully and during 15 months of follow-up none had relapsed.[19]

The search for perfection in chemotherapy had not yet ended and the next move originated in Hong Kong where the tuberculosis problem had been tackled with energy and determination. There, by 1973, an effectively supervised out-patient treatment scheme was in being, starting with a phase of daily dosage and continuing with the usual twice weekly isoniazid plus streptomycin programme. Mindful of the practical benefits of short-course chemotherapy which could be intermittent from the start, the Hong Kong Tuberculosis Treatment Services, in conjunction with the British Medical Research Council, elected to study further the streptomycin-isoniazid-pyrazinamide combination which had been used in East Africa. The participants in the trial were divided into three groups: one group received all three drugs daily and their progress was compared with that of the other two groups who were receiving the same drugs (but with a higher dosage of isoniazid and of pyrazinamide) three times weekly and twice weekly respectively for either 6 months or 9 months, the exact duration being decided by random allocation. All three drugs were given together under direct supervision. Following the termination

17   Brouet, G. & Roussel, G. (1974) Modalités et bilan des traitements courts. p. 27 XVIIe Congrès National de la Tuberculose & des Maladies Respiratoires. Clermont-Ferrand.
18   Poppe de Figueiredo, P. et al. (1974) Short duration chemotherapy of pulmonary tuberculosis: a pilot trial. Proc. XXIInd. Int. Tuberc. Conf. *Bull. int. Un. Tuberc.* 49, 382.
19   British Thoracic & Tuberculosis Association (1975) Short-course chemotherapy in pulmonary tuberculosis. *Tubercle 56*, 165.

of treatment at six months the relapse rate during the subsequent six months was 13 per cent of those on the daily regimen 16 per cent on the thrice weekly and 18 per cent on the twice weekly. When treatment had been continued for nine months relapse occurred in 3 per cent who had been on daily chemotherapy and 4 per cent in each of the other two groups. All those patients who relapsed did so with fully sensitive organisms and the vast majority of relapses occurred within three months of ceasing treatment.[20]

It is clear that the last word on chemotherapy has not yet been said and that short-course treatment may fulfill the hopes of its sponsors and provide a fresh and more flexible approach to the whole management of the disease. More investigation is still required to determine precisely those factors—drug combinations, dosage rhythms, length of treatment—required to achieve the twin targets of complete therapeutic efficiency and patient acceptability. These two ends are mutually interdependent and although they have not yet been attained it would indeed be a man of little faith who would now deny that such attainment may well be successfully accomplished before the passing of the present decade.

20 Fox, W. & Mitchison, D. A. (14).

Chapter Twenty-one
The Last Frontier

Never in the long history of tuberculosis had there been any period to bear comparison with the 30 years that followed Waksman's discovery—30 years of high drama and revolutionary change that had seen the wonders of the past, artificial pneumothorax and pneumoperitoneum, swept into oblivion together with the mutilating crudities of the surgery of pulmonary tuberculosis, so recently hailed as the ultimate in therapeutic endeavour. By the early 1970s intensive research work, backed in many instances by the financial resources of the major pharmaceutical firms, had produced such a sufficiency and variety of antibacterial agents that it had become possible to offer a guarantee of cure to any patient with tuberculosis—provided that the agents were correctly employed.

The control of tuberculosis now became an attainable objective: even its eradication was no longer just a pipe-dream, though the world had still to appreciate that mere acquisition of the means of eliminating tuberculosis was not enough. The weapons available had to be utilized effectively and in accordance with an overall strategic plan in the formulation of which the kindred disciplines of epidemiology and immunology, sociology and medical administration had to stand shoulder to shoulder with clinical therapeutics.

In Britain the dawn of the chemotherapeutic era had coincided with the genesis of the National Health Service in 1948 and the planning of the latter created an opportunity to eliminate some of the more obvious defects in the scheme for tuberculosis which had been initiated and perpetuated by the implementation of the Astor Report of 1912. The illogical separation of tuberculosis from general medicine and surgery had long been recognized as an administrative misfortune as had also the patchwork quality of the service resulting from the variation in size and in financial strength of the controlling local authorities. Under the new plan the latter were relieved of all

243

responsibilities for the diagnosis and treatment of tuberculosis which became a charge upon the 19 recently created Regional Hospital Boards although arrangements for the prevention of the disease and for the social welfare of its victims were, somewhat anomalously, to remain with the local authorities.

The result of this change in the structure of administration led gradually towards the forging and strengthening of links between the general hospitals and the sanatoria and such a process of integration once begun, had a wholly beneficial effect upon the tuberculosis service. The erstwhile sanatoria were gradually upgraded into chest hospitals, the tuberculosis dispensaries were expanded and re-equipped, becoming chest clinics which were frequently re-sited in juxtaposition to the medical outpatient departments of the general hospitals, while the tuberculosis officers were invested with the title of chest physicians and eventually admitted to the exclusive hierarchy of hospital consultants which had hitherto been the preserve of the general physicians.

As evidence of the potency of antituberculosis chemotherapy accumulated the pace of change accelerated. A departmental scheme was drawn up for the closure or transfer to other use of redundant chest hospitals while an official brake was put upon recruitment into the speciality of chest medicine by a sharp reduction in the number of junior training posts within the service. These remarkable happenings must have suggested to the public that tuberculosis had indeed been vanquished and that the whole somewhat distasteful subject—for despite large sums spent on popular enlightenment the social stigma attaching to a diagnosis of 'consumption' had never been wholly eliminated—could now be handed over to the medical historians. Such facile optimism was generated solely in the minds of the ad-ministrators and was never shared by the clinicians who, dealing daily with realities, saw that while methods might be changing tuberculosis still remained a serious problem and that the ground which had been gained could readily be lost again if the attack was not pressed home. The rapid rundown of the service which had appeared imminent was only stayed when an influx of immigrants from high prevalence areas brought a sharp reminder that any relaxation of vigilance or curtail-ment of facilities must keep pace with events and not outrun them.

In the United States there was less haste to dismantle the machinery which had been created and, although this led in some instances to the retention of traditional procedures beyond the point when they had outlived their usefulness, such a cautiously conservative approach on the part of the responsible authorities was understandable rather than blameworthy.

Tuberculosis as a global problem had, at an early stage, engaged the interest and attention of the World Health Organisation and, in accordance with its general policy of convening groups of international experts to advise on technical and scientific matters, it proceeded to set up an Expert Committee on Tuberculosis. When this Committee held its seventh meeting, in 1960, it reported that tuberculosis was 'generally conceded to be the most important specific communicable disease in the world as a whole, and its control should receive priority and emphasis both by WHO and by governments'.[1]

In 1964 the Committee reviewed the progress which had been made and in its subsequent report a note of disappointment was clearly discernible.

> The Committee noted that the specific tools now available for preventing and curing tuberculosis made it possible to plan and execute effective antituberculosis programmes under practically any epidemiological or socio-economic conditions. It stressed that the relatively slow decline in the tuberculosis problem observed in many countries seems to be in contrast to the resources expended on tuberculosis programmes, and that localized increases in incidence have even occurred recently in several developed countries. The Committee thought that this unsatisfactory situation is due mainly to insufficient realism in selecting priorities for application; lack of national planning, co-ordination and evaluation; and failure to re-orient traditional approaches to present knowledge. Particularly there seems to be inadequate recognition that an efficient tuberculosis control programme depends upon reliable epidemiological and operational data, permitting its continuous adaptation to changing circumstances.[2]

Having voiced this criticism the Committee then devoted much of the remainder of its Report to the provision of constructive and practical advice designed to guide those charged with the planning and organization of national tuberculosis campaigns.

Ten years later, in 1974, the WHO Expert Committee published its Ninth Report, which opened with a reminder from Dr M. Takabe,

1 World Health Organisation (1960) WHO Expert Committee on Tuberculosis. *Tech. Rep. Series 195*, 4.
2 World Health Organisation (1964) WHO Expert Committee on Tuberculosis. *Tech. Rep. Series 290*, 3–4.

Director of the Organisation's Division of Communicable Diseases, that tuberculosis still remained a major problem in all the developing countries:

> In some areas of Africa, Asia and Oceania the reported annual incidence of pulmonary tuberculosis is 200–350 cases per 100 000 inhabitants and the prevalence is usually at least twice as high. The number of infectious cases of tuberculosis in the world at present is estimated to be in the range of 15–20 millions. Tuberculosis also remains a problem in many technically advanced countries: in countries where it is considered rare, it often causes more deaths than all other notifiable infectious diseases combined.[3]

In debating the reasons for this failure in achievement the Committee, after reiterating its belief that the principles laid down at the 1964 meeting still retained their validity, stated that unfortunately many problems had been encountered in the implementation of the suggested programme.

> Shortages of financial, material and physical resources and a shortage or maldistribution of trained manpower are aggravated by a lack of managerial skill ... In some countries a major constraint has been a reluctance to change traditional and outmoded orientations. Determined leadership is needed to effect the necessary changes and to apply more effectively the potent measures available for tuberculosis control.[4]

In the main body of the Report the Committee once again set out the requirements for a successful world campaign. They stressed the need for a basic structure of adequate epidemiological data and added a reminder that the indices on which reliance had been placed in the past now lacked authority. The introduction of chemotherapy had deprived mortality figures of much of their former significance, save that a high mortality rate was a clear indication of an inadequate programme, while notification figures as currently reported were either inaccurate or incomplete and therefore constituted no true index of actual epidemiological trends. It was suggested that both these indices be discarded and replaced by two others which the Committee held to be more relevant to the measurement of the extent

3 World Health Organisation (1974) WHO Expert Committee on Tuberculosis. *Tech. Rep. Series 552*, 5.
4 *Ibid.* 6.

of the tuberculosis problem in a community and hence to the strategy of programme planning:

(a) the prevalence of tuberculosis patients excreting tubercle baccilli demonstrable by direct smear examination—such patients are mainly responsible for the transmission of infection and the disease in the community; (b) the age-specific prevalence of tuberculous infection as demonstrated by tuberculin testing.[5]

After discussing the techniques of predictive epidemiology and surveillance the Report went on to express satisfaction over the increasing use of BCG vaccination and to commend the action of WHO in establishing an international control system to ensure that all vaccine utilized was of the highest quality.

In an important section devoted to case-finding and treatment the Committee stressed the vital point that the former was not an end in itself but merely the preliminary to treatment and cure. Consequently it was essential to ensure that any expansion of a case-finding programme was not permitted to outstrip the capacity of the service to provide effective chemotherapy for the patients. The abandonment of mass radiography as an indiscriminate means of case-finding was recommended both on grounds of expense and of the demands which this method made on the services of highly qualified technicians and medical staff who could be employed to better purpose in other public health activities. The following practical methods of screening were considered to offer the best prospects:

(1) the examination of patients who present themselves with relevant symptoms to any health facility, (2) increasing the awareness of the community, the medical profession and all cadres of staff involved in the programme concerning the importance of symptoms referable to the respiratory system . . . especially if they have been present for more than four weeks, (3) the examination of contacts, especially if they have symptoms, (4) the bacteriological examination of patients who have had a radiographic examination of the chest for whatever reason, if it shows a lesion with a possible tuberculous etiology, (5) the examination of immigrants and foreign workers coming from high prevalence areas—the Committee strongly recommends that their treatment should be the responsibility of the host country.[6]

5   *Ibid.* 7.
6   *Ibid.* 15.

Much stress was laid upon the importance of bacteriological examination in establishing a definitive diagnosis, the Committee pointedly remarking that when chemotherapy was initiated on the basis of radiographic findings alone a substantial proportion of patients were treated unnecessarily.

In the section of the Report which dealt with treatment full emphasis was placed on adequate chemotherapy:

> Such treatment meets the expressed needs of the patients who present with symptoms and saves many lives ... chemotherapy should be available, free of cost, for every patient detected. In the developing countries widespread treatment services may be feasible only if careful attention is paid to the rational utilization of the available funds and health personnel.[7]

In its advocacy of adequate chemotherapy for all requiring it the Committee reiterated a previous recommendation that 'the financial resources and manpower available for tuberculosis control be used to organize efficient and widespread ambulatory programmes rather than to support hospital treatment'; and, noting with concern the adherence to outmoded long-term sanatorium treatment in some technically advanced countries, urged the national authorities thereof to 'review the reasons for the retention of traditional sanatorium services despite the dramatic progress of chemotherapy in the last 20 years'.

In commenting upon the drug regimens appropriate for a national campaign the Committee drew heavily upon the work and experience of the Madras Centre, singling out for special comment the proven benefits of an initial period of triple drug therapy and the very considerable advantages to be gained from a directly supervised intermittent regimen. Short-course regimens of six months or thereabouts were regarded as being still at the experimental stage but there was support for the view that the 18 month to two year course, accepted as standard in many countries, was unnecessarily long and that it should prove more rewarding to concentrate on ensuring that each patient continued with treatment for one year without interruption.

As a corollary to the more general availability of increasingly potent antituberculosis drugs and the advances made in their employment the Committee supported the view already gaining ground in

7 *Ibid.* 17.

Britain[8] and in some areas of the United States,[9] that the traditional prolonged follow-up of patients who had completed an adequate course of chemotherapy was unnecessary. Relapse in modern circumstances should be very rare and the time and resources previously expended on follow-up clinics could be used to better purpose in improving supervision of the original chemotherapy. Reassurance was also offered on the problem of initial drug resistance, that possible sequel to acquired resistance which had caused so much anxiety to physicians everywhere. Visualized originally as a problem which was likely to increase over the years, studies in Britain had already provided evidence that the feared increase was not materializing and now, as the result of studies over a wider area, the WHO Report was encouraging:

> The Committee emphasized that the importance of initial drug resistance as a cause of treatment failure has been much overrated. Failure to respond to the standard regimens of chemotherapy because of initial drug resistance is more likely to occur in patients with strains resistant to two or all three of the drugs in the regimen than in those with resistance to one strain only. Patients with multiple-drug-resistant strains, however, represent only a very small proportion of the total even in communities in which drug resistance is known to be common.[10]

Finally, in the concluding section of the Report, the Committee reiterated the conviction of its members that

> since reliable diagnostic tools and efficacious preventive (BCG) and curative (chemotherapy) methods are available and because they can be both simple and inexpensive, the control of tuberculosis deserves a high priority on the list of rewarding health programmes. An effective national tuberculosis programme can be delivered under any situation, provided planning and application are guided by a clear understanding of the epidemiological, technical, operational, economic and social aspects.[11]

This admirable report, compiled by acknowledged experts and refreshingly free from the grinding of political axes, provided a succinct and lucid account of the progress which had been made in

---

8   Horne, N. W. (1966) Chronic pulmonary tuberculosis. Present problems. *Bull. int. Un. Tuberc. 37*, 172.
9   Edsall, J. & Collins, G. (1973) Routine follow-up of inactive tuberculosis. A practice to be abandoned. *Am. Rev. resp. Dis. 107*, 851.
10   World Health Organisation (3) 20–1.
11   *Ibid.* 22.

the international campaign against tuberculosis. Clearly much had been found to criticize in the campaign as then conducted, but the criticism was constructive and the Committee rightly believed that it had a duty to provide guidance on the framing of any programme designed to secure the elimination of tuberculosis as a significant communicable disease. Much of the guidance was presented with the needs of countries with limited resources clearly in mind; but the problem in the economically more fortunate differs only in its extent and in the ease with which facilities can be mobilized. A concerted and sustained effort by the more affluent nations, based upon the precepts laid down by this WHO Committee, should be capable of bringing their own tuberculosis problem under control and leave them free to play an increasingly worthwhile part in the global campaign by giving all possible assistance to those areas which are less lavishly endowed.

Waksman and his successors have supplied the world with the weapons with which the eradication of tuberculosis can be accomplished. It would be but a poor return for their brilliance and their dedication if the world, through default, inertia or political manoeuvring, were to prove itself incapable of using these weapons to the full.

Indexes

Names

Where several references appear under a name the most important are indicated in bold type.

Names

General

*Where several references appear under an entry
the most important are indicated in bold type.*

A

Academy of Medicine, Paris   47, 49, 55,
  58
After-care
  definition   129
  farm colony   129, 144, 150
  village settlement   145, 150, 151
  vocational training   144, 150, 151
Alcohol   *see* Therapy
Alexandrian School of Medicine   8, 12
Altitude   *see* Therapy
Altro workshops   145–6
American Association for Thoracic
  Surgery   174
American Medical Association   63, 114
Anatomical studies of Galen   14
  corrected by Vesalius   20
'Antiphlogistic' therapy   *see* Therapy
Apicolysis   *see* Pneumonolysis,
  extrapleural
Arabian medicine   52
Artificial pneumothorax
  Carson's principles   105–6
  case selection   160, 163
  early attempts   106, 107, 110, **111–14,**
    115–19
  Forlanini's priority conceded   117
  Medical Research Council Report
    158–9
  pleural adhesions   106, 113, **120–2,**
    126, 159, **160–2,** 168
    see also Pneumonolysis, intrapleural
  results   162–3
  'selective' collapse   120
  simultaneous bilateral collapse   119–20
  water manometer   117–18
Asklepieia   6–7
Antituberculosis schemes **128–30, 134–40,**
  151, 152–5, 181, 245, **246–8,** 249
  local authorities   129, 132–3, 134, 137,
    152–3, 154–6, 244

Astor Committee and Report   130, **134–6,**
  143, 151, 152–3, 154, 156, 188, 243
  see also Tuberculosis, Departmental
    Committee *and* Report on, 1912
Autopsies, lack of   8, 20
Ayur–Veda   *see* Indo–Aryan medicine

B

Babylonian medicine   1–2
Bacille Calmette-Guerin (BCG)
  discovery   189–90
  vaccine   190–200
    conflicting results   196–7
    criticism of Calmette   191–2
    developing countries   200, 247, 249
    Lubeck disaster   192
    mass vaccination   *see* International
      Tuberculosis Campaign
    Medical Research Council's
      controlled trial   195–6
    non-specific mycobacterial infection
      198, 201
    safety   190, 192
    Scandinavia   193–4
    United Kingdom   194–6
    United States   191, 196–9
      editorial in *American Review of
        Respiratory Disease*   198
      letter in *British Medical Journal*   197
      safety queried   191, 197
    World Health Organisation   199,
      247, 249
Barlow Committee and Report   *see*
  Inter-Departmental Committee on
  Tuberculosis (Sanatoria for Soldiers)
Bellevue Hospital   62, 175
Berlin Physiological Society   60
Bleeding   *see* Therapy, venesection